Mechanical Ventilation

A short course on the
theory and application
of mechanical ventilators

Robert L. Chatburn, BS, RRT-NPS, FAARC

Director
Respiratory Care Department
University Hospitals of Cleveland
Associate Professor
Department of Pediatrics
Case Western Reserve University
Cleveland, Ohio

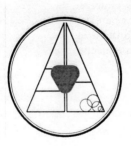

Mandu Press Ltd.
Cleveland Heights, Ohio

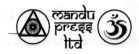

Published by:
Mandu Press Ltd.
PO Box 18284
Cleveland Heights, OH   44118-0284

First Edition

Copyright © 2003 by Robert L. Chatburn

Library of Congress Control Number: 2003103281

ISBN, printed edition: 0-9729438-2-X

ISBN, PDF edition: 0-9729438-3-8

First printing: 2003

Table of Contents

Table of Figures

Table of Tables

Preface

Find a better way to educate students than the current books offer. If you can't improve on what's available, what's the point?

Earl Babbbie
Chapman University

This book is about how ventilators work. It shows you how to think about ventilators, when to use various modes, and how to know if they are doing what you expect. This book does not say much about how to use ventilators in various clinical situations or how to liberate patients from the machine. Mechanical ventilation is still more of an art than a science. This book leads you to expertise with the theory and tools of that art. You will then be able to make the best use of other books and actual clinical experience.

There are 18 books devoted to mechanical ventilation on my bookshelf. They are all well written by noted experts in the field. Some are commonly used in colleges while others have fallen into obscurity. Yet, in my opinion, they all have the same limitation; they devote only a small fraction of their pages to how ventilators actually work. Most of their emphasis is on how ventilators are used to support various disease states, the physiological effects of mechanical ventilation, weaning, and adjuncts like artificial airways and humidifiers. This book is different.

The reason I made this book different may be clarified by analogy. Suppose you wanted to learn how to play the guitar. You go to the library, but all you can find are books that give you a few pages describing what different guitars look like and all the fancy names and features their manufacturers have made up. There may be a little information about how many strings they have and even what notes and chords can be played. Unfortunately, many of the books use words with apparently conflicting or obscure meanings. There is no consistency and no music theory. They all devote most of their content to a wide variety of song scores, assuming the few pages of introduction to the instrument will allow you to play them. How well do you think you would learn to play the guitar from these books? If you have ever actually tried it, you would see the difficulty. That approach works for a simple instrument like a harmonica, but it does not work well for a complex device like a mechanical ventilator. In a similar fashion, we don't let our teenagers drive cars after simply pointing out the controls on the dashboard; they have to sit through weeks of theory before ever getting behind the wheel.

You can kill or injure somebody with a ventilator just as fast as you can with a car.

Certainly there is a great need for understanding the physiological effect of mechanical ventilation. But most authors seem to put the cart before the horse. In this book, I have tried to present the underlying concepts of mechanical ventilation from the perspective of the ventilator. All terminology has been clearly defined in a way that develops a consistent theoretical framework for understanding how ventilators are designed to operate. There is one chapter devoted to how to use ventilators, but it is written from the perspective of what the ventilator can do and how you should think about the options rather than from what physiological problem the patient may have. There is also a chapter devoted to monitoring the ventilator-patient interface through waveform analysis, a key feature on modern ventilators. In short, this book will teach you how to think about ventilators themselves. It teaches you how to master the instrument. That way you are better prepared to orchestrate patient care. Only after thoroughly understanding what ventilators do will you be in a position to appreciate your own clinical experience and that of other expert authors.

The unique approach of this book makes it valuable not only to health care workers but to those individuals who must communicate with clinicians. This includes everyone from the design engineer to the marketing executive to the sales force and clinical specialists. Indeed, since manufacturers provide most of the education on mechanical ventilation, the most benefit may come from advancing their employees' level of understanding.

How to Use This Book

This book may be read on a variety of levels depending on your educational needs and your professional background. Look at the different approaches to reading and see what is most appropriate for you.

Basic Familiarity: This level is appropriate for people not directly responsible for managing ventilators in an intensive care environment. This may include healthcare personnel such as nurses, patients on home care ventilators, or those not directly involved at the bedside such as administrators or ventilator sales personnel. Study the first two chapters and the section on alarms in Chapter 3. Skim the others for areas of interest, paying attention to the figures in Chapter 5.

Comprehensive Understanding: Respiratory care students should achieve this level along with physicians and nurses who are responsible for ventilator management. Some sales personnel may wish to understand ventilators at this level in order to converse easily with those who buy and use them. Study all the chapters, but skip the "Extra for Experts" sections. Pay attention to the "Key Idea" paragraphs and the definitions in the Glossary. Make sure you understand Chapter 5.

Subject Mastery: This level is desirable for anyone who is in a position to teach mechanical ventilation and particularly for those who are involved with research on the subject. All material in the book should be understood, including the "Extra for Experts" sections. A person at this level should be able to answer all the questions and derive all the equations used throughout.

Of course, these levels are only suggestions and you will undoubtedly modify them for your own use.

———

Acknowledgement

The central ideas of this text came from two seminal papers I published in Respiratory Care, the official scientific journal of the American Association for Respiratory Care. The first was published in 1991, and introduced a new classification system for mechanical ventilators (Respir Care 1991:36(10):1123-1155). It was republished the next year as a part of the Journal's Consensus Conference on the Essentials of Mechanical Ventilators (Respir Care 1992:37(9):1009-1025). Eventually, those papers became the basis for book chapters on ventilator design in every major respiratory care textbook:

- Tobin MJ. *Principles and Practice of Mechanical Ventilation*, 1994. McGraw-Hill.

- Branson RD, Hess DR, Chatburn RL. *Respiratory Care Equipment*, 1st and 2nd editions, 1995 & 1999. Lippincott.

- White GC. Equipment for Respiratory Care 2nd edition, 1996, Delmar.

- Hess DR, Kacmarek RM. *Essentials of Mechanical Ventilation*, 1996. McGraw-Hill.

- Pilbeam SP. Mechanical Ventilation. Physiological and Clinical Applications, 3rd edition, 1998. Mosby.

- Scanlan CL, Wilkins RL, Stoller JK. *Egan's Fundamentals of Respiratory Care* 7th edition, 1999. Mosby.

- Branson RD. MacIntyre NR. *Mechanical Ventilation*, 2001. WB Saunders.

- Wyka KA, Mathews PJ, Clark WF. *Foundations of Respiratory Care*, 2002. Delmar.

- Hess DR, MacIntyre NR, Mishoe SC, Galvin WF, Adams WB, Saposnick AB. *Respiratory Care. Principles and Practice*, 2002. Saunders.

In 2001, my coauthor, Dr. Frank Primiano Jr., and I introduced a new system for classifying modes of ventilation (Respir Care 2001; 46(6):604-621), tying in with the principles established in the earlier publications. That paper received the Dr. Allen DeVilbiss Technology Paper Award for best paper of the year at the 2001 International Respiratory Care Congress. Only the last book listed above has that information.

In this book you are getting the latest information, undiluted, uninterpreted, from the original author.

Dedication

It's an endless, glamorless, thankless job.
But somebody's got to do it.

Sergeant Joe Friday
LAPD

This book is dedicated to everyone who has ever tried to teach the subject of mechanical ventilation. It has always been a daunting task, given the lack of a unified lexicon, complex technological advances, and an endless stream of clinical studies and conflicting opinions. Yet, here and there, lone educators stay up endless nights writing textbooks and lectures; intrepid clinical specialists fly red-eye specials around the globe to eager but clueless audiences; sales personnel valiantly argue their cause; and frustrated engineers try to communicate with inventive clinical researchers. Much of this effort is expended simply for the love of the subject. Keep up the good work; you benefit countless lives.

1. INTRODUCTION TO VENTILATION

During breathing, a volume of air is inhaled through the airways (mouth and/or nose, pharynx, larynx, trachea, and bronchial tree) into millions of tiny gas exchange sacs (the alveoli) deep within the lungs. There it mixes with the carbon dioxide-rich gas coming from the blood. It is then exhaled back through the same airways to the atmosphere. Normally this cyclic pattern repeats at a breathing rate, or frequency, of about 12 breaths a minute (breaths/min) when we are at rest (a higher resting rate for infants and children). The breathing rate increases when we exercise or become excited.[1]

Gas exchange is the function of the lungs that is required to supply oxygen to the blood for distribution to the cells of the body, and to remove carbon dioxide from the blood that the blood has collected from the cells of the body. Gas exchange in the lungs occurs only in the smallest airways and the alveoli. It does not take place in the airways (conducting airways) that carry the gas from the atmosphere to these terminal regions. The size (volume) of these conducting airways is called the **anatomical dead space** because it does not participate directly in gas exchange between the gas space in the lungs and the blood. Gas is carried through the conducting airways by a process called "convection". Gas is exchanged between the pulmonary gas space and the blood by a process called "diffusion".

Key Idea

> One of the major factors determining whether breathing is producing enough gas exchange to keep a person alive is the ventilation the breathing is producing. Ventilation (usually referred to as **minute ventilation**) is expressed as the volume of gas entering, or leaving, the lungs in a given amount of time. It can be calculated by multiplying the volume of gas, either inhaled or exhaled during a breath (called the **tidal volume**), times the breathing rate (for example: 0.5 Liters x 12 breaths/min = 6 L/min).

---

[1] This section is adapted from: Primiano FP Jr, Chatburn RL. What is a ventilator? Part I. www.VentWorld.com; 2001.

> The level of ventilation can be monitored by measuring the amount of carbon dioxide in the blood. For a given level of carbon dioxide produced by the body, the amount in the blood is inversely proportional to the level of ventilation.

Therefore, if we were to develop a machine to help a person breathe, or to take over his or her breathing altogether, it would have to be able to produce a tidal volume and a breathing rate which, when multiplied together, produce enough ventilation, but not too much ventilation, to supply the gas exchange needs of the body. During normal breathing the body selects a combination of a tidal volume that is large enough to clear the dead space and add fresh gas to the alveoli, and a breathing rate that assures the correct amount of ventilation is produced. However, as it turns out, it is possible, using specialized equipment, to keep a person alive with breathing rates that range from zero (steady flow into and out of the lungs) up to frequencies in the 100's of breaths per minute. Over this frequency range, convection and diffusion take part to a greater or lesser extent in distributing the inhaled gas within the lungs. As the frequency is increased, the tidal volume that produces the required ventilation gets smaller and smaller.

There are two sets of forces that can cause the lungs and chest wall to expand: the forces produced when the muscles of respiration (diaphragm, inspiratory intercostal, and accessory muscles) contract, and the force produced by the difference between the pressure at the airway opening (mouth and nose) and the pressure on the outer surface of the chest wall. Normally, the respiratory muscles do the work needed to expand the chest wall, decreasing the pressure on the outside of the lungs so that they expand, which in turn enlarges the air space within the lungs, and draws air into the lungs. The difference between the pressure at the airway opening and the pressure on the chest wall surface does not play a role in this activity under normal circumstances. This is because both of these locations are exposed to the same pressure (atmospheric), so this difference is zero. However, when the respiratory muscles are unable to do the work required for ventilation, either or both of these two pressures can be manipulated to produce breathing movements, using a mechanical ventilator.

It is not difficult to visualize that, if the pressure at the airway opening (the mouth and nose or artificial airway opening) of an individual were increased while the pressure surrounding the rest of the person's body remained at atmospheric, the person's chest would expand as air is literally forced into the lungs. Likewise, if the pressure on the person's body surface were lowered as the pressure at the person's open mouth and nose remained at atmospheric, then again the pressure at the mouth would be greater than that on the body surface and air would be forced into the lungs.

Key Idea

Thus, we have two approaches that can be used to mechanically ventilate the lungs: apply positive pressure (relative to atmospheric) to the airway opening - devices that do this are called **positive pressure ventilators**; or, apply negative pressure (relative to atmospheric) to the body surface (at least the rib cage and abdomen) - such devices are called **negative pressure ventilators**.

Sometimes positive airway pressure is applied to a patient's airway opening without the intent to ventilate but merely to maintain a normal lung volume. Originally, devices were designed to present resistance to expiratory flow, and hence provide positive pressure throughout expiration. The pressure at end expiration was called positive end expiratory pressure or **PEEP**. The problem with these early devices was that the patient had to inhale with enough force to drop the airway pressure through the PEEP level to below atmospheric pressure before inspiratory flow would begin. This often increased the work of breathing to intolerable levels. Newer devices were designed to avoid this problem. The key was to design the device so that the patient could inspire by dropping the pressure just below the PEEP level, rather than all the way to atmospheric pressure. As a result, the pressure in the patient's lungs remained positive (above atmospheric) throughout the breathing cycle. Thus, the new procedure was called continuous positive airway pressure or **CPAP**. Almost all current ventilators provide CPAP rather than PEEP. There are also devices that just produce CPAP for patients that are breathing without a ventilator.

As time passed, people forgot the historic reasons for the distinction between PEEP and CPAP. The original PEEP therapy is now called "positive airway pressure", PAP, and is used to help patients (who are not connected to mechanical ventilators) to mobilize airway secretions and reverse atelectasis. Currently, the term PEEP is applied to the continuous positive airway pressure provided during assisted ventilation by a mechanical ventilator. Assisted ventilation means simply that the ventilator helps the patient with the timing and/or work of inspiration. The term CPAP is usually applied to continuous positive airway pressure provided while the patient breathes unassisted, such as for infants with respiratory distress syndrome after extubation or adults with sleep apnea.

It is important to remember that CPAP and PEEP themselves are not forms of assisted ventilation, in the sense that they do not supply any of the work of breathing. They may, however, make it easier for the patient to breathe by lowering airway resistance or increasing lung compliance.

Self Assessment Questions

Definitions

Explain the meaning of the following terms:

- Anatomical dead space
- Minute ventilation
- Tidal volume
- PEEP
- CPAP

True or False

1. Gas exchange is the function of the lungs that is required to supply oxygen to the blood for distribution to the cells of the body, and to remove carbon dioxide from the blood that the blood has collected from the cells of the body.

2. Gas exchange occurs in all the conducting airways and the alveoli.

3. Minute ventilation is calculated as the product of tidal volume and breathing rate.

4. The unit of measurement for minute ventilation is liters.

5. It is possible to keep a person alive with breathing rates that range from zero (steady flow into and out of the lungs) up to frequencies in the 100's of breaths per minute.

Multiple Choice

1. The forces that expand the lungs and chest wall during inspiration are:

   a. The forces produced when the muscles of respiration (diaphragm, inspiratory intercostal, and accessory muscles) contract.

   b. Positive end expiratory pressure (PEEP).

   c. The force produced by the difference between the pressure at the airway opening (mouth and nose) and the pressure on the outer surface of the chest wall.

   d. Both a and c.

2. In order to generate an inspiration, the following condition must be present:

   a. Lung pressure must be higher than pressure at the airway opening.

   b. Airway pressure must be higher than body surface pressure.

   c. Body surface pressure must be higher than airway pressure.

   d. Pleural pressure must be lower than body surface pressure.

3. In order to generate an expiration, the following condition must be present:

   a. Lung pressure must be higher than pressure at the airway opening.

   b. Pressure at the airway opening must be higher than body surface pressure.

   c. Body surface pressure must be higher than pressure at the airway opening.

   d. Body surface pressure must be lower than lung pressure.

Key Ideas

1. What two variables determine whether breathing is producing enough gas exchange to keep a person alive?

2. Explain how the level of ventilation can be monitored by measuring carbon dioxide in the blood. Why not just measure tidal volume and frequency?

3. Describe the difference between positive pressure ventilators and negative pressure ventilators.

2. INTRODUCTION TO VENTILATORS

A mechanical ventilator is an automatic machine designed to provide all or part of the work the body must produce to move gas into and out of the lungs. The act of moving air into and out of the lungs is called breathing, or, more formally, ventilation.

The simplest mechanical device we could devise to assist a person's breathing would be a hand-driven, syringe-type pump that is fitted to the person's mouth and nose using a mask. A variation of this is the self-inflating, elastic resuscitation bag. Both of these require one-way valve arrangements to cause air to flow from the device into the lungs when the device is compressed, and out from the lungs to the atmosphere as the device is expanded. These arrangements are not automatic, requiring an operator to supply the energy to push the gas into the lungs through the mouth and nose. Thus, such devices are not considered mechanical ventilators.

Automating the ventilator so that continual operator intervention is not needed for safe, desired operation requires:

- a stable attachment (interface) of the device to the patient,

- a source of energy to drive the device,

- a control system to regulate the timing and size of breaths, and

- a means of monitoring the performance of the device and the condition of the patient.

Types of Ventilators

We will consider two classes of ventilators here. First are those that produce breathing patterns that mimic the way we normally breathe. They operate at breathing rates our bodies normally produce during our usual living activities: 12 - 25 breaths/min for children and adults; 30 - 40 breaths/min for infants. These are called **conventional ventilators** and their maximum rate is 150 breaths/minute.[1] Second are those that produce breathing patterns at frequencies much higher than we would or could voluntarily produce for breathing - called **high frequency ventilators**. These ventilators can produce rates up to 15 Hz (900 breaths/minute).

Conventional Ventilators

The vast majority of ventilators used in the world provide conventional ventilation. This employs breathing patterns that approximate those produced by a normal spontaneously breathing person. Tidal volumes are large enough to clear the anatomical dead space during inspiration and the breathing rates are in the range of normal rates. Gas transport in the airways is dominated by convective flow and mixing in the alveoli occurs by molecular diffusion. This class of ventilator is used in the ICU, for patient transport, for home care and in the operating room. It is used on patients of all ages from neonate to adult.

High Frequency Ventilators

It has been known for several decades that it is possible to adequately ventilate the lungs with tidal volumes smaller than the anatomic dead space using breathing frequencies much higher than those at which a person normally breathes. This is actually a common occurrence of which we may not be fully aware. Dogs do not sweat. They regulate their temperature when they are hot by panting as you probably know. When a dog pants he takes very shallow, very fast, quickly repeated breaths. The size of these panting breaths is much smaller than the animal's anatomical dead space, especially in dogs with long necks. Yet, the dog feels no worse for this type of breathing (at least all the dogs interviewed for this article).

Devices have been developed to produce high frequency, low amplitude breaths. These are generally used on patients with respiratory distress syndrome, whose lungs will not expand properly. These are most often neonates whose lungs have not fully developed, but can also be older patients whose lungs have been injured. High frequency ventilators are also used on patients that have lungs that leak air. The very low tidal volumes produced put

---

[1] This is a limit imposed by the Food and Drug Administration on manufacturers.

less stress on fragile lungs that may not be able to withstand the stretch required for a normal tidal volume.

There are two main types of high frequency ventilators: **high frequency jet ventilators (HFJV)** and **high frequency oscillatory ventilators (HFOV)**. The HFJV directs a high frequency pulsed jet of gas into the trachea from a thin tube within an endotracheal or tracheostomy tube. This pulsed flow entrains air from inside the tube and directs it toward the bronchi. The HFOV typically uses a piston arrangement (although other mechanisms are used) that moves back and forth rapidly to oscillate the gas in the patient's breathing circuit and airways. Both of these techniques cause air to reach the alveoli and carbon dioxide to leave the lungs by enhancing mixing and diffusion in the airways. Convection plays a minor role in gas transport with these ventilators while various forms of enhanced diffusion predominate.

Although high frequency devices that drive the pressure on the chest wall have been developed, most high frequency ventilators in use today are applied to the airway opening.

Patient-Ventilator Interface

Positive Pressure Ventilators

The ventilator delivers gas to the patient through a set of flexible tubes called a **patient circuit**. Depending on the design of the ventilator, this circuit can have one or two tubes.

Key Idea

> The circuit connects the ventilator to either an endotracheal or tracheostomy tube that extends into the patient's throat (causing this arrangement to be called **invasive ventilation**), or a mask covering the mouth and nose or just the nose (referred to as **noninvasive ventilation**).

Each of these connections to the patient may have a balloon cuff associated with it to provide a seal - either inside the trachea for the tracheal tubes or around the mouth and nose for the masks.

Negative Pressure Ventilators

The patient is placed inside a chamber with his or her head extending outside the chamber. The chamber may encase the entire body except for the head (like the iron lung), or it may enclose just the rib cage and abdomen (chest cuirass). It is sealed to the body where the body extends outside the chamber. Although it is not generally necessary, the patient may have an endotracheal or tracheostomy tube in place to protect the airway from aspiration.

Power Source

Positive Pressure Ventilators

Positive pressure ventilators are typically powered by electricity or compressed gas. Electricity is used to run compressors of various types. These provide compressed air for motive power as well as air for breathing. More commonly, however, the power to expand the lungs is supplied by compressed gas from tanks, or from wall outlets in the hospital. The ventilator is generally connected to separate sources of compressed air and compressed oxygen. This permits the delivery of a range of oxygen concentrations to support the needs of sick patients. Because compressed gas has all moisture removed, the gas delivered to the patient must be warmed and humidified in order to avoid drying out the lung tissue. A humidifier placed in the patient circuit does this. A humidifier is especially needed when an endotracheal or tracheostomy tube is used since these cover or bypass, respectively, the warm, moist tissues inside of the nose and mouth and prevent the natural heating and humidification of the inspired gas.

Negative Pressure Ventilators

Negative pressure ventilators are usually powered by electricity used to run a vacuum pump that periodically evacuates the chamber to produce the required negative pressure. Humidification is not needed if an endotracheal tube is not used. Oxygen enriched inspired air can be provided as needed via a breathing mask.

Control System__

A control system assures that the breathing pattern produced by the ventilator is the one intended by the patient's caregiver. This requires the setting of control parameters such as the size of the breath, how fast and how often it is brought in and let out, and how much effort, if any, the patient must exert to signal the ventilator to start a breath.

Key Idea

> If the patient can control the timing and size of the breath, it is called a **spontaneous** breath. Otherwise, it is called a **mandatory** breath. This distinction is important because it is the basis for defining a mode of ventilation. A **mode** of ventilation is a particular pattern of spontaneous and mandatory breaths.

Numerous modes, with a variety of names, have been developed to make ventilators produce breathing patterns that coordinate the machine's activity with the needs of the patient

Patient Monitoring System

Most ventilators have at least a pressure monitor (measuring airway pressure for positive pressure ventilators, or chamber pressure for negative pressure ventilators) to gauge the size of the breath and whether or not the patient is properly connected to the ventilator. Many positive pressure ventilators have sophisticated pressure, volume and flow sensors that produce signals both to control the ventilator's output (via feedback in the ventilator's control system) and to provide displays (with alarms) of how the ventilator and patient are interacting. Clinicians use such displays to follow the patient's condition and to adjust the ventilator settings.

Alarms

All but the most simple transport ventilators have some type of alarm system to warn the operator of malfunctions or dangerous patient situations. We will describe alarms in detail in the next chapter. For now, it is enough to know that there are three basic types of alarms (1) input power alarms, (2) control circuit alarms, and (3) output alarms.

Input power alarms warn of disconnection of the ventilator from its electrical or pneumatic power source. Most such alarms are battery operated but in some cases, they may be pneumatic. For example, if the oxygen source becomes disconnected, the air source may power a pneumatic alarm.

Control circuit alarms do two things: warn of electronic control circuit failures and alert the operator to incompatible ventilator settings. An example of the incompatible settings might be that the inspiratory time is set too high compared to the rate.

Output alarms indicate that the pressure, volume, or flow generated during ventilation of the patient is outside safe or expected limits. In addition, there are usually alarms for inspired gas temperature and oxygen concentration.

Graphic Displays

Modern ICU ventilators provide graphic displays in two formats: **waveforms** (sometimes called scalars) and **loops**. Waveform displays show pressure, volume, and flow on the vertical axis with time on the horizontal axis. Loop displays show one variable plotted against another. Chapter 5 gives a detailed explanation of how graphic displays are interpreted. However, we will review the basics here so that you will be comfortable with some of the figures in the next two chapters.

Waveform Displays

The ideal waveform display allows you to view pressure, volume, and flow waveforms all at the same time, or in any combination. Some ventilators allow only two variables to be displayed at a time, in which case pressure and flow give the most information. Figure 2-1 illustrates the ideal display with some points of interest.

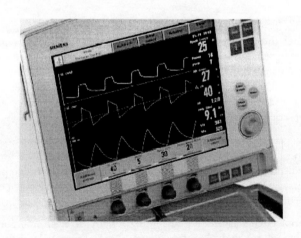

Figure 2-1. A display of pressure, volume, and flow waveforms during mechanical ventilation.

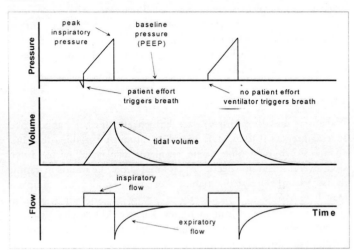

Loop Displays

There are two common loop displays used to assess patient-ventilator interactions. One shows volume on the vertical axis and pressure on the horizontal axis. This type of loop allows you to see the effects of compliance and resistance. The other common display shows flow on the vertical axis and volume on the horizontal axis. This loop is typically used to assess the need for, and effects of, bronchodilators on airways resistance. Figure 2-2 illustrates these two types of loops.

Figure 2-2. Two types of loops commonly used to assess patient-ventilator interactions.

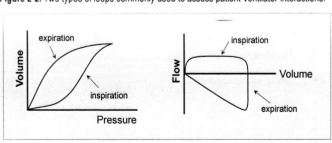

Calculated Parameters

Some ventilators are capable of calculating various physiologic parameters such as estimates of respirator system mechanics such as resistance, compliance and work of breathing. They may even calculate indices such as the mean airway pressure and minute ventilation. Some ventilators will display values derived from separate devices such as end tidal carbon dioxide monitors. Calculated values will be described in detail in Chapter 5.

Trends

Waveform and loop displays are limited events that happen over several breaths. Often, it is useful to monitor variables that may change slowly over time. Some ventilator displays allow for a very slow sweep speed on special displays that show the trends in various measured and calculated variables over long periods. For example, it may be possible to plot the mean airway pressure or respiratory system compliance over many hours. This would be helpful to track the increase or decrease in ventilatory support and the course of the patient's disease.

Self Assessment Questions

Definitions

- Mechanical ventilator

- Conventional ventilator

- High frequency ventilator

- High frequency jet ventilator

- High frequency oscillatory ventilator

- Spontaneous breath

- Mandatory breath

- Mode of ventilation

- Waveform display

- Loop display

True or False

1. A manual resuscitation bag is considered a mechanical ventilator.

2. High frequency ventilators typically deliver tidal volumes that are less than the anatomical dead space.

3. Two types of noninvasive ventilators are the iron lung and the chest cuirass. The iron lung encases the whole body except for the head while the chest cuirass covers only the rib cage and abdomen.

4. An artificial airway is necessary to perform noninvasive ventilation.

5. Positive pressure ventilators are typically used with some type of humidifier.

Multiple Choice

1. All of the following types of breaths are classified as mandatory except:

    a. The patient starts and stops the breath.

    b. The patient starts the breath but the ventilator stops it.

    c. The ventilator starts the breath but the patient stops it.

    d. The ventilator starts and stops the breath.

2. Humidifiers are used during invasive mechanical ventilation for all the following reasons except:

    a. Compressed gas is dry.

    b. The nose, which would normally supply heat and humidity, is bypassed by the artificial airway.

    c. To reduce the risk of retained secretions.

    d. To filter the gas of dust particles.

3. Ventilator monitors perform all of the following functions except:

    a. Alert the operator if the patient becomes disconnected.

    b. Control the size and frequency of the breath.

    c. Display pressure, volume, and flow waveforms.

    d. Allow the operator to assess how well the ventilator interacts with the patient.

Key Ideas

1. What is the difference between invasive and noninvasive ventilation? What is the correlation between positive and negative pressure ventilators?

2. Why is the distinction between spontaneous and mandatory breath types important?

*"**Health Devices** has repeatedly stressed the need for users to understand the operation and features of ventilators, regardless of whether they will be used to ventilate neonatal/pediatric or adult patients. The fact that ventilators are such an established technology by no means guarantees that these issues are clearly understood...we continue to receive reports of hospital staff misusing ventilators because they're unaware of the devices' particular operational considerations."*

ECRI Health Devices July 2002, Volume 31, Number 7

3. HOW VENTILATORS WORK

If you want to understand how ventilators work, and not just how to turn the knobs, it is essential to have some knowledge of basic mechanics. We begin by recognizing that a ventilator is simply a machine designed to transmit applied energy in a predetermined manner to perform useful work. Ventilators are powered with energy in the form of either electricity or compressed gas. That energy is transmitted (by the ventilator's drive mechanism) in a predetermined manner (by the control circuit) to assist or replace the patient's muscular effort in performing the work of breathing (the desired output). Thus, to understand ventilators we must first understand their four mechanical characteristics:

1) Input power

2) Power conversion and transmission

3) Control system

4) Output (pressure, volume, and flow waveforms)

We can expand this simple outline to add as much detail about a given ventilator as desired. A much more detailed description of ventilator design characteristics can be found in books on respiratory care equipment.[1]

---

[1] Branson RD, Hess DR, Chatburn RL. Respiratory Care Equipment, 2nd Ed. Philadelphia: Lippencott Williams & Wilkins, 1999.   ISBN 0-7817-1200-9

Input Power

The power source for a ventilator is what generates the force to inflate the patient's lungs. It may be either electrical energy (Energy = Volts × Amperes × Time) or compressed gas (Energy = Pressure × Volume). An electrically powered ventilator uses AC (alternating current) voltage from an electrical line outlet. In addition to powering the ventilator, this AC voltage may be reduced and converted to direct current (DC). This DC source can then be used to power delicate electronic control circuits. Some ventilators have rechargeable batteries to be used as a back-up source of power if AC current is not available.

A pneumatically powered ventilator uses compressed gas. This is the power source for most modern intensive care ventilators. Ventilators powered by compressed gas usually have internal pressure reducing valves so that the normal operating pressure is lower than the source pressure. This allows uninterrupted operation from hospital piped gas sources, which are usually regulated to 50 p.s.i. (pounds per square inch) but are subject to periodic fluctuations.

Power Transmission and Conversion

The power transmission and conversion system consists of the drive and output control mechanisms. The drive mechanism generates the actual force needed to deliver gas to the patient under pressure. The output control consists of one or more valves that regulate gas flow to and from the patient.

The ventilator's drive mechanism converts the input power to useful work. The type of drive mechanism determines the characteristic flow and pressure patterns the ventilator produces. Drive mechanisms can be either: (1) a direct application of compressed gas through a pressure reducing valve, or (2) an indirect application using an electric motor or compressor.

The output control valve regulates the flow of gas to and from the patient. It may be a simple on/off exhalation. An example would be the typical infant ventilator. The valve in the exhalation manifold closes to provide a periodic pressure waveform that rises to a preset limit during inspiration (forcing gas into the lungs) then opens to allow pressure to fall to another preset limit during exhalation (allowing gas to escape from the lungs). Alternatively, there can be a set of output control valves that shape the output waveform. An example would be the Hamilton Galileo ventilator. This ventilator uses an exhalation manifold valve that closes to force gas into the lungs or opens to allow exhalation. There is also a flow control valve that shapes the inspiratory flow waveform once the exhalation manifold closes.

Control System

The Basic Model of Breathing (Equation of Motion)

We use models of breathing mechanics to provide a foundation for understanding how ventilators work. These models simplify and illustrate the relations among variables of interest. Specifically, we are interested in the pressure needed to drive gas into the airway and inflate the lungs.

The physical model of breathing mechanics most commonly used is a rigid flow conducting tube connected to an elastic compartment as shown in Figure 3-1. This is a simplification of the actual biological respiratory system from the viewpoint of pressure, volume, and flow.

The mathematical model that relates pressure, volume, and flow during ventilation is known as the **equation of motion** for the respiratory system:

muscle pressure + *ventilator pressure* = *(elastance × volume)* + *(resistance × flow)*

This equation is sometimes expressed in terms of compliance instead of elastance.

muscle pressure + *ventilator pressure* = *(volume/ compliance)* + *(resistance × flow)*

Pressure, volume and flow are variable functions of time, all measured relative to their end expiratory values. Under normal conditions, these values are: muscle pressure = 0, ventilator pressure = 0, volume = functional residual capacity, flow = 0. During mechanical ventilation, these values are: muscle pressure = 0, ventilator pressure = PEEP, volume = end expiratory volume, flow = 0. Elastance and resistance are constants.

When airway pressure rises above baseline (as indicated by the ventilator's airway pressure display), inspiration is assisted. The pressure driving inspiration is called **transrespiratory system pressure**. It is defined as the pressure at the airway opening (mouth, endotracheal tube or tracheostomy tube) minus the pressure at the body surface. Transrespiratory system pressure has two components, **transairway pressure** (defined as airway opening pressure minus lung pressure) and **transthoracic pressure** (defined as lung pressure minus body surface pressure). We may occasionally use the term **transpulmonary pressure**, defined as airway opening pressure minus pleural pressure.

Figure 3-1. Models of the ventilatory system. P = pressure. Note that compliance = 1/elastance. Note that intertance is ignored in this model, as it is usually insignificant.

Key Idea

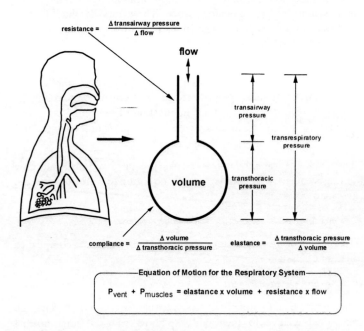

$$\text{resistance} = \frac{\Delta \text{transairway pressure}}{\Delta \text{flow}}$$

flow

transairway pressure

transrespiratory pressure

volume

transthoracic pressure

$$\text{compliance} = \frac{\Delta \text{volume}}{\Delta \text{transthoracic pressure}} \qquad \text{elastance} = \frac{\Delta \text{transthoracic pressure}}{\Delta \text{volume}}$$

Equation of Motion for the Respiratory System

$$P_{vent} + P_{muscles} = \text{elastance} \times \text{volume} + \text{resistance} \times \text{flow}$$

Muscle pressure is the imaginary (unmeasurable) transrespiratory system pressure generated by the ventilatory muscles to expand the thoracic cage and lungs. Ventilator pressure is transrespiratory system pressure generated by the ventilator. The combined muscle and ventilator pressures cause gas to flow into the lungs.

Elastance (elastance = Δpressure/Δvolume) together with **resistance** (resistance = Δpressure/Δflow) contribute to the load against which the muscles and ventilator do work (note that load has the units of pressure, so the left side of the equation equals the right side).

So the equation of motion may also be expressed as:

muscle pressure + ventilator pressure = elastic load + resistive load

Elastic load is the pressure required to deliver the tidal volume (elastance times tidal volume) and **resistive load** is the pressure required to deliver the flow (resistance times flow). Note: it is sometimes more convenient to speak of compliance instead of elastance. **Compliance** is defined as Δvolume/Δpressure and is equal to 1/elastance.

Key Idea

> From the equation, we see that if ventilator pressure is zero, the muscles provide all the work of breathing. This is normal, unassisted breathing. Note that if the patient is connected to a ventilator and the ventilator provides exactly the flow demanded by the patient's inspiratory effort, the airway pressure will not rise above baseline ($P_{vent} = 0$ throughout inspiration). If the ventilator does not provide enough flow to meet the demand, airway pressure will fall below baseline. On the other hand, if the ventilator provides more flow than is demanded by the patient, then airway pressure will rise above baseline and inspiration is said to be "assisted". If both the muscle pressure and the ventilator pressure are non-zero, the patient provides some of the work and the ventilator provides some work. This is called **partial ventilatory support**. If the muscle pressure is zero, the ventilator must provide all the work of breathing. This is called **total ventilatory support**.

Review and Consider

1. The equation of motion for the respiratory system can be traced to Newton's Third Law of Motion: Every action has an equal and opposite reaction. In fact, the equation of motion is sometimes called a "force balance" equation. Why? (*Hint: what is the unit of measurement that results from multiplying elastance by resistance or multiplying resistance by flow?*)

2. Rewrite the equation of motion in using only transrespiratory pressure, transthoracic pressure and transairway pressure.

3. Write the equation of motion for unassisted spontaneous inspiration and for assisted ventilation of a paralyzed patient.

4. Write the equation of motion for passive expiration.

5. If lung elastance increases, what happens to lung compliance?

6. Use the equation of motion to show what happens to airway pressure if airway resistance decreases during mechanical ventilation.

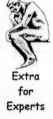

Extra
for
Experts

The model shown in Figure 3-1 is really an oversimplification of the actual respiratory system. For example, it lumps together chest wall and lung compliance as well as lumping together the compliances of the two lungs. In addition, it lumps together the resistances of all the many airways. It also ignores inertance (the constant of proportionality between pressure and the rate of change of flow) because the inertia of the gas, lungs, and chest wall are insignificant at normal frequencies.

For some discussions, it is more useful to have multi-compartment models. To simplify the drawing of such models, we borrow symbols from electrical engineering. Specifically, a resistor in electronics is used to represent airway resistance and a capacitor is used to represent compliance. The ventilator may be represented as a constant voltage source (a pressure controller) as shown in Figure 3-1 or it may be represented as a constant current source (a flow controller). Figure 3-2 shows a multi-compartment model using electrical components.

In Figure 3-2, the trachea is connected in series with the right and left mainstem bronchi, which are connected to each other in parallel. In addition, the right and left lungs are connected in parallel and the two are connected in series with the chest wall. We can also add the resistance and compliance of the patient circuit.

Figure 3-2. Multi-compartment model of the respiratory system connected to a ventilator using electronic analogs. Note that the right and left lungs are modeled as separate series connections of a resistance and compliance. However, the two lungs are connected in parallel. The patient circuit resistance is in series with the endotracheal tube. The patient circuit compliance is in parallel with the respiratory system. The chest wall compliance is in series with that of the lungs. The function of the exhalation manifold can be shown by adding a switch that alternately connects the patient and patient circuit to the positive pole of the ventilator (inspiration) or to ground (the negative pole, for expiration). Note that inertance, modeled as an electrical inductor, is ignored in this model as it is usually negligible.

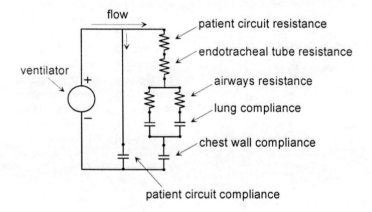

What do we mean by series and parallel connections? This is terminology borrowed from electrical engineering. A **series connection** means that two or more components share the same flow but each has a different pressure drop (the pressure difference between inlet and outlet). An example would be an endotracheal tube in series with the mainstem bronchus. The total resistance of a series connection is just the sum of the individual resistances. Another example of a series connection is the elastance of the lungs and the chest wall. The total elastance of a series connection is again the sum of the individual elastances. However, the total compliance (reciprocal of elastance) of a series connection is calculated as

$$\frac{1}{C_{total}} = \frac{1}{C_1} + \frac{1}{C_2}$$

This equation can be rearranged to give:

$$C_{total} = \frac{C_1 \times C_2}{C_1 + C_2}$$

Note that while the total series resistance or elastance is greater than that of any component, the total series compliance is *less than* the compliance of any component.

A **parallel connection** means that two or more components share the same pressure drop but different flows. An example would be the resistances of the right and left bronchi. Resistances in parallel act like compliances in series; they add reciprocally. Therefore, the total resistance of a parallel connection of resistances is less than the resistance of either component. The same is true for elastances. However, compliances in parallel add like resistances in series; they are summed together. Thus, the total compliance of the right and left lungs connected in parallel is greater than the compliance of either lung.

Series and parallel connections are illustrated in Figure 3-3.

Series Connection

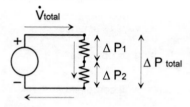

Parallel Connection

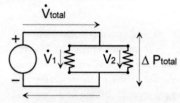

Figure 3-3. Series and parallel connections using electronic analogs. $\dot{V}$ = flow, P = pressure

All this talk about series and parallel connections may seem irrelevant now, but you will see its importance in Chapter 5 when we discuss how changes in respiratory system mechanics affect graphic displays of pressure, volume, and flow.

Later, we will have occasion to talk about lung damage due to mechanical ventilation. In that context, it is helpful to identify the components of transthoracic pressure as **transalveolar pressure**

(pressure inside the lung or alveoli minus pleural pressure) and **transmural pressure** (pleural pressure minus body surface pressure.

Thus,

$$P_{transrespiratory} = P_{transairway} + P_{transthoracic} = P_{transairway} + (P_{transalveolar} + P_{transmural})$$

From this you can see that the pressure displayed by the ventilator is affected by the mechanical properties of the airways, the lungs, and the chest wall.

You may have noticed by now that the structures we have been modeling are in fact *defined* by the locations of the pressure measurements. For example, the respiratory system is everything that exists between the two locations where *transrespiratory pressure* is measured (the airway opening and the body surface). Similarly, the pulmonary system is defined by the *transpulmonary pressure* points (airway opening and pleural space). The airways are everything between the points used for defining *transairway pressure* (airway opening and inside the lungs). The thoracic system lies between the points used for *transthoracic pressure* (inside the lungs and body surface). *Transalveolar pressure* defines the alveoli (lungs) as existing between the inside of the lungs and the pleural space. Finally, the chest wall lies between the points for *transmural pressure* (pleural space and body surface). A model of some portion of the respiratory system can be represented by adding the component pressures. For example, for the pulmonary system:

$$P_{transpulmonary} = P_{transairway} + P_{transalveolar.}$$

Knowledge of how these models fit together is helpful in understanding the mechanics of ventilation, how different modes work, and for creating research simulations.

Control Circuit

The ventilator must have a control circuit to manipulate pressure, volume, and flow. The control circuit measures and directs the output of the ventilator. It may include mechanical, pneumatic, electric, electronic, or fluidic components. Most modern ventilators combine two or more of these subsystems to provide user control.

Mechanical control circuits use devices such as levers, pulleys, and cams. These types of circuits were used in the early manually operated ventilators illustrated in history books. Pneumatic control is provided using gas-powered pressure regulators, needle valves, jet

Mechanical Ventilation

entrainment devices, and balloon-valves. Some transport ventilators use pneumatic control systems.

Electric control circuits use only simple switches, rheostats (or potentiometers), and magnets to control ventilator operation. Electronic control circuits use devices such as resistors, capacitors, diodes, and transistors as well as combinations of these components in the form of integrated circuits. The most sophisticated electronic systems use microprocessors to control ventilator function.

Some transport ventilators use fluidic logic control circuits. These are pneumatic circuits that function much like electrical circuit boards. Fluidic control mechanisms have no moving parts. In addition, fluidic circuits are immune to failure from surrounding electromagnetic interference, as can occur around MRI equipment.

Control Variables

A **control variable** is the primary variable that the ventilator control circuit manipulates to cause inspiration.

Key Idea

> There are only three variables in the equation of motion that a ventilator can control: pressure, volume, and flow. Because only one of these variables can be directly controlled at a time, a ventilator must function as either a pressure, volume, or flow controller.

Time is implicit in the equation of motion and in some cases will serve as a control variable. Figure 3-4 illustrates the criteria for determining the control variable.

Figure 3-4. The criteria for determining the control variable during mechanical ventilation.

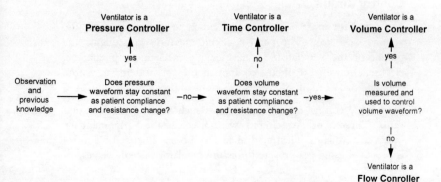

Pressure

If the ventilator controls pressure, the pressure waveform will remain unchanged with changes in respiratory system mechanics but volume and flow will vary. The ventilator can control either the airway pressure (causing it to rise above body surface pressure for inspiration) or the pressure on the body surface (causing it to fall below airway opening pressure for inspiration). This is the basis for classifying ventilators as being either positive or negative pressure types. ⎯⎯

Volume

If the ventilator controls volume, the volume and flow waveforms will remain unchanged with changes in respiratory mechanics but pressure will vary. To qualify as a true volume controller, a ventilator must measure volume and use this signal to control the ventilator output (the volume waveform). Volume can be controlled directly by the displacement of a device such as a piston or bellows. Volume can be controlled indirectly by controlling flow.

Flow

If the ventilator controls flow, the flow and volume waveforms will remain unchanged with changes in respiratory mechanics but pressure will vary. Flow can be controlled directly using something as simple as a flow meter or as complex as a proportional solenoid valve. Flow can be controlled indirectly by controlling volume.

Review and Consider

7. Explain how the equation of motion relates to classifying ventilator control variables.

8. What type of pattern would you expect to see on a ventilator graphics display when a ventilator is operating as a pressure controller? What waveform would you look at first, pressure, volume, or flow?

9. Suppose you observe on a graphics monitor that a ventilator always delivers a constant inspiratory flow. What else must you know to determine the control variable?

Phase Variables

A complete cycle or breath controlled by a ventilator consists of four phases:

1) starting inspiration,

2) inspiration itself,

3) ending inspiration,

4) expiration.

To understand a breath cycle, you must know how the ventilator starts, sustains, and stops inspiration and you must know what occurs between breaths.

The **phase variable** is a signal that is measured and used by the ventilator to initiate some part, or phase, of the breath cycle.

Key Idea

> The variable causing a breath to begin is the **trigger variable**. A variable whose magnitude is constrained to some maximum value during inspiration is called a **limit variable**. The variable causing a breath to end is the **cycle variable**. During expiration, the ventilator usually maintains some level of pressure at or above atmospheric pressure (positive end expiratory pressure, or PEEP), which is referred to as the **baseline variable**.

Trigger Variable

A breath can be initiated by either the machine or the patient. If the machine initiates the breath, the trigger variable is time. If the patient initiates the breath, pressure, flow, or volume may serve as the trigger variable. Manual or operator-initiated triggering is also available on most ventilators. Some ventilators provide other ways of detecting the patient's inspiratory effort and thus triggering inspiration. Examples of other trigger variables include esophageal pressure, chest wall motion, and thoracic impedance.

Once the trigger variable signals the start of inspiration, there is always a short delay before flow to the patient starts. This delay is called the **response time** and is due to signal processing time and the mechanical inertia of the drive mechanism. It is important for the ventilator to have a short response time to maintain optimal synchrony with the patient's inspiratory effort.

Time Triggering

Time triggering means that inspiratory flow starts because a preset expiratory time interval has elapsed.

There are several time intervals of interest during expiration. One is the **expiratory flow time**. Gas travels from the patient to the atmosphere during this time. Another interval is the **expiratory pause time**, during which expiratory flow has ceased but inspiratory flow has not yet started. An expiratory hold is sometimes imposed (by intentionally interrupting expiratory flow) to measure autoPEEP. The sum of the expiratory flow time and the expiratory **pause time** is the **expiratory time**. This is illustrated in Figure 3-5.

Figure 3-5. Time intervals of interest during expiration.

y Idea

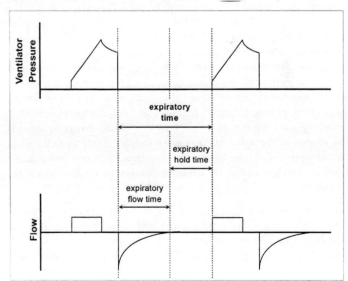

Time triggering is usually associated with the ventilator's rate control. Specific systems for setting a breathing rate vary from ventilator to ventilator. The most common approach is a rate or frequency (breaths per minute) control. When a rate control is used, inspiratory and expiratory times will vary according to other control settings, such as flow and volume. An alternative approach is to provide separate timers for inspiration and expiration. Changing either or both of these timers will alter the frequency (see discussion under *Time Cycling*).

Patient Triggering

With patient triggering, the ventilator must "sense" the patient's effort. This is usually done by measuring either airway pressure or flow, although other variables may be used. As the patient makes an inspiratory effort, the value of the trigger variable changes. The **sensitivity** setting of the ventilator is the threshold value for the trigger variable which, when met, starts inspiration.

Pressure triggering occurs when a patient's inspiratory effort causes a drop in pressure within the patient circuit. When this pressure drop reaches the preset sensitivity threshold, inspiration triggers on and gas delivery begins. On most ventilators, you can adjust the pressure drop needed to trigger a breath. Typically, you set the sensitivity 0.5 to 1.5 cm H_2O below the baseline expiratory pressure. Setting the trigger level to a higher number, say 3.0 cm H_2O, makes the ventilator less sensitive and requires the patient to work harder to initiate inspiration. Conversely, setting the trigger level lower makes the ventilator more sensitive. This convention comes from the engineering definition of sensitivity; a change in output divided by a given change in input. In this case, the change in output is switching from expiration to inspiration and the change in input is the change in the value of the trigger variable (such as a change in airway pressure). Thus, the smaller the change in the denominator (the trigger variable), the larger the ratio and the greater the sensitivity.

Using flow as the trigger variable is a bit more complex. Typically, the ventilator provides a continuous low flow of gas through the patient circuit. The ventilator measures the flow coming out of the main flow control valve and the flow through the exhalation valve. If the patient is motionless, these two flows are equal (assuming no leaks in the patient circuit). When the patient makes an inspiratory effort, the flow through the exhalation valve falls below the flow from the output valve as flow is diverted into the patient's lungs. The difference between these two flows is the flow trigger variable.

To adjust the sensitivity of a flow-triggered system, you usually set both a base continuous flow and a flow trigger threshold. Typically, the trigger threshold is set at 1 to 3 L/min (below baseline). For example, if you set the base continuous flow at 10 L/min and the trigger at 2 L/min, the ventilator will trigger when the flow at the exhalation manifold falls to 8 L/min or less. An alternative approach used by some ventilators is to simply measure the flow at the wye connector[2] and trigger on that signal.

Theoretically, flow triggering imposes less work on the patient than pressure triggering. Imposed work to trigger is proportional to the volume of gas the patient must inspire from the patient circuit and the resulting pressure drop. With pressure triggering, the pressure drop depends on the sensitivity setting; so imposed work is always present. With flow triggering, the pressure drop is very small no matter what the sensitivity setting; so imposed work tends to be less.

One ventilator, the Dräger Babylog, uses inspired volume as a trigger signal. The volume signal is obtained by integrating the flow signal using a sensor at the airway opening. The theoretical advantage of using volume is that integration reduces the noise in the flow signal and thereby potentially reduces triggering errors.

Limit Variable

To **limit** means to restrict the magnitude of a variable. A **limit variable** is one that can reach and maintain a preset level *before* inspiration ends but does not end inspiration. Pressure, flow, or volume can be the limit variable, and can actually all be set as limit variables for a single breath (e.g. using the P_{max} feature on a Dräger ventilator).

Clinicians often confuse limit variables with cycle variables. To **cycle** means to end inspiration. A cycle variable always ends inspiration. A limit variable does not terminate inspiration; it only sets an upper bound for pressure, volume, or flow (see Figure 3-6).

The confusion over limit and cycle variables is due, in part, to the nomenclature used by many ventilator manufacturers. They often

---

[2] The connector that joins the inspiratory and expiratory limbs of the patient circuit with the endotracheal tube.

use the term limit to describe what happens when a pressure or time alarm threshold is met (that is, inspiration is terminated and an alarm is activated). To be consistent with accepted nomenclature, it is best to refer to these alarm thresholds as backup cycling mechanisms rather than limits.

Figure 3-6. The importance of distinguishing between the terms *limit* and *cycle*. A. Inspiration is pressure limited and time cycled. B. Flow is limited but volume is not, and inspiration is volume cycled. C. Both volume and flow are limited and inspiration is time cycled.

Key Idea

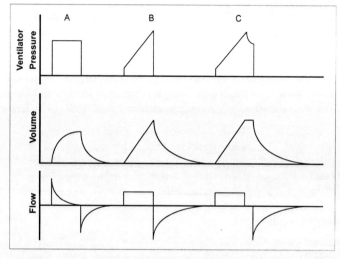

There is another confusing issue regarding pressure limits. On most ventilators, the pressure limit for mandatory breaths is measured relative to atmospheric pressure. However, when a spontaneous breath is assisted with pressure (eg, Pressure Support mode) the pressure limit is measured relative to the baseline (PEEP) pressure. For example, if PEEP is 5 cm H_2O and the Pressure Support level is 10 cm H_2O, the peak inspiratory pressure would be 15 cm H_2O (above atmospheric pressure).

Cycle Variable

The inspiratory phase always ends when some variable reaches a preset value. The variable that is measured and used to end inspiration is called the **cycle variable**. The cycle variable can be pressure, volume, flow, or time. Manual cycling is also available on some ventilators.

Pressure Cycling

When a ventilator is set to pressure cycle, it delivers flow until a preset pressure is reached. When the set pressure is achieved, inspiratory flow stops and expiratory flow begins. The most common application of pressure cycling is for alarm settings.

Volume Cycling

When a ventilator is set to volume cycle, it delivers flow until a preset volume has passed through the control valve. By definition, as soon as the set volume is met, inspiratory flow stops and expiratory flow begins. If expiration does not begin immediately after inspiratory flow stops, then an inspiratory hold has been set and the ventilator is, by definition, time cycled (see below). Note that the volume that passes through the ventilator's output control valve is never exactly equal to the volume delivered to the patient because of the volume compressed in the patient circuit. Some ventilators use a sensor at the wye connector (like the Dräger Evita 4 with the neonatal circuit) for accurate tidal volume measurement. Others measure volume at some point inside the ventilator and the operator must know whether the ventilator compensates for compressed gas in its tidal volume readout.

Flow Cycling

When a ventilator is set to flow cycle, it delivers flow until a preset level is met. Flow then stops and expiration begins. The most frequent application of flow cycling is in the Pressure Support mode. In this mode, the control variable is pressure and the ventilator provides the flow necessary to meet the inspiratory pressure limit. In doing so, flow starts out at a relatively high value and decays exponentially. Once flow has decreased to a relatively low value (such as 25% of peak flow, typically preset by the manufacturer) inspiration is cycled off. Manufactures often set the cycle threshold slightly above zero flow to avoid inspiratory times from getting so long that patient synchrony is degraded. On some ventilators, the flow cycle threshold may be adjusted by the operator to improve patient synchrony.

Time Cycling

Time cycling means that expiratory flow starts because a preset inspiratory time interval has elapsed.

There are several time intervals of interest during inspiration (Figure 3-7). One is the **inspiratory flow time**. Gas travels from the ventilator to the patient during this time. Another interval is the **inspiratory pause time**, during which inspiratory flow has ceased but expiratory flow is not yet allowed. An inspiratory hold is sometimes set on the ventilator (Figure 3-7) to determine the static lung pressure so that compliance can be calculated, or simply to hold the lungs open longer in an attempt to improve oxygenation. The sum of the inspiratory flow time and the inspiratory pause time is the **inspiratory time**. Time cycling occurs when the inspiratory time has elapsed.

Figure 3-7. Time intervals of interest during inspiration. Note that pressure drops from peak to static (plateau) value during the inspiratory hold.

Key Idea

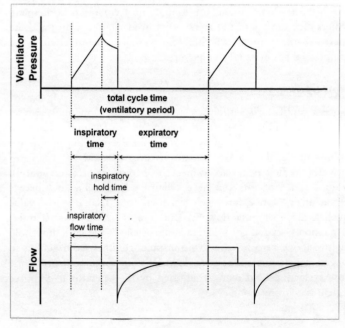

Now that we have defined both inspiratory time and expiratory time, we can define the **total cycle time** as the sum of the two. This is also called the **ventilatory period** (measured in seconds) and is related to ventilatory frequency (*f*, in cycles per minute) as follows:

$$f = \frac{1}{period} = \frac{60 \text{ seconds}}{T_\text{I} + T_E}$$

where inspiratory time, T_I and expiratory time T_E are both measured in seconds. Changing T_I or T_E changes frequency. For example, if inspiratory time is increased, the ventilatory period (or total cycle time) is increased and frequency is decreased.

Inspiratory times and expiratory times are related to each other through the I:E ratio:

$$I : E = \frac{T_I}{T_E}$$

Alternatively, some ventilators use duty cycle or percent inspiration:

$$\% \ inspiration = \frac{T_I}{T_I + T_E} \times 100\% = \frac{I}{I+E} \times 100\%$$

The percent inspiration is easily converted into the I:E ratio:

$$I : E = (\% \ inspiration) : (100\% - \% \ inspiration)$$

For example, an I:E ratio of 1:2 is a duty cycle of 33% and a duty cycle of 50% represents an I:E ratio of 1:1.

Machine versus Patient Cycling

When talking about modes, it is sometimes more convenient to say that a breath is either machine cycled or patient cycled, rather than describe the exact cycle variable. To be patient cycled, the patient must be able to change the inspiratory time by making either inspiratory or expiratory efforts. If this is not possible, then the breath is, by definition, machine cycled. For example, with pressure cycling, the patient can make the inspiratory time longer by making an inspiratory effort. Because the patient is breathing in, it takes longer for the ventilator to generate the set pressure. (From the ventilator's point of view, it looks like the patient's compliance has greatly increased.) The patient can shorten inspiratory time by making an expiratory effort, forcing the pressure to rise more rapidly. Another example of patient cycling is the Pressure Support mode. Here, inspiration ends when flow decays to some preset value. Just as with pressure cycling, the patient can either prolong or shorten the time to the threshold flow. If the ventilator is time cycled, it is by definition machine cycled, as the patient cannot do anything to change the inspiratory time aside from getting out of bed and turning a knob. Volume cycling is usually a form of machine cycling. That is because all ventilators today deliver the preset volume at a preset flow, and this determines the inspiratory time (inspiratory time = volume/flow). If a ventilator was designed to allow the patient to draw as much flow as needed but still cycle when the preset volume was delivered, then this type of volume cycling could be patient cycling because the patient could shorten inspiratory time by making an inspiratory effort. This is not likely to happen because no designer would allow the patient to get more flow and then arbitrarily stop inspiration in the middle of an effort.

In summary, time and volume cycling are typically referred to as "machine cycling" while pressure and flow cycling are types of "patient cycling".

Review and Consider

10. What are the four phases of a breath delivered by a mechanical ventilator?

11. Why must there be a defined phase variable for the ventilator's control circuit to operate?

12. What does expiratory time have to do with the start of inspiration and ventilatory frequency?

13. What are the two components of expiratory time?

14. In what clinical situation might you want to create an expiratory hold?

15. What are the two components of inspiratory time?

16. If inspiratory time is 1 second and expiratory time is 2 seconds. What is the ventilatory frequency? Calculate the I:E ratio and duty cycle.

17. Is an I:E ratio of 1:2 larger or smaller than a ratio of 1:3?

18. Suppose the control variable is flow. What would the volume waveform look like if inspiratory time was longer than inspiratory flow time?

19. Suppose a ventilator is flow limited and volume cycled. If you create an inspiratory hold, have you changed the limit or cycle variables?

20. If a breath is volume limited, what would you expect to see on the graphic waveform display?

Baseline Variable

The baseline variable is the parameter controlled during expiration. Although pressure, volume, or flow could serve as the baseline variable, pressure control is the most practical and is implemented by all modern ventilators.

Baseline or expiratory pressure is always measured and set relative to atmospheric pressure. Thus, when we want baseline pressure to equal atmospheric pressure, we set it to zero. When we want baseline pressure to exceed atmospheric pressure, we set a positive value, called positive end-expiratory pressure (PEEP).

Recall from Chapter 1 our discussion about the difference between PEEP and CPAP. We said that PEEP generally refers to baseline pressure during mechanical ventilation while CPAP usually refers to spontaneous breathing, although technically, it is all CPAP. However, the point I want to make here is that there are different ways of controlling airway pressure.

The simplest way to create CPAP would be to pinch off the end of a straw so that it had a high resistance. That resistance would create backpressure as you exhale through the straw. Such a system is actually used to provide PEP (positive expiratory pressure) therapy to spontaneously breathing patients in order to treat atelectasis and improve mucus removal. The problem is that the pressure level depends on the expiratory flow. Thus, it is not a very good system for ventilating patients who cannot be expected to cooperate.

A better way of obtaining a PEEP effect is to connect the expiratory tubing to a container of water. Imagine exhaling through a straw whose end is submerged 5 centimeters below the surface of a glass of water. The pressure in your airways while you exhale would be about 5 centimeters of water pressure. This technique has actually been used clinically, especially in creating CPAP for infants. The CPAP effect can be simulated with a spring-loaded valve, which is still used on some ventilators. The main advantage of this type of system is that airway pressure stays relatively constant regardless of flow.

Of course, the most accurate way to create CPAP would be to connect the straw to some sort of electronic valve that measured the CPAP level and automatically adjusted the expiratory resistance to maintain a steady pressure level regardless of the flow. This is how most modern ventilators do it. Figure 3-8 illustrates the pressure waveforms expected with these three types of expiratory pressure devices

These techniques differ in another way. What happens if the patient inhales while connected to the device? In the first case, the patient would inhale, cause the airway pressure to drop, yet get no air because water simply goes up the straw (Figure 3-8 A). In the second case, the patient inhales, causes the airway pressure to drop, and gets a limited flow of air through the restriction (Figure 3-8 B). In the last case, if the electronic valve is sophisticated enough, the patient inhales, the valve opens, and there is little or no drop in pressure as she gets all the air she wants (Figure 3-8 C).

Here is the interesting thing: Ventilator manufacturers created the first electronic PEEP valves for ventilators decades ago. But they failed to realize that patients might make inspiratory efforts on their own during what the ventilator thought was expiratory time. The result was the effect shown in Figure 3-8 A, where the patient tries to inhale but gets no flow. This results in an increased work of breathing and discomfort for the patient. Eventually, exhalation valves were created that let the patient breathe spontaneously while maintaining the set CPAP level. Years later, pressure controlled ventilation of adults became popular. Valves were created that could generate one level of constant pressure during inspiration and then drop back to the CPAP level during expiration. Unfortunately, manufacturers made the same mistake about inspiration in that they failed to accommodate the possibility that the patient might try to inhale during the mandatory inspiratory time. Again, the effect was like that shown in Figure 3-8 A. More years passed and finally, today, manufacturers use valves that work like Figure 3-8 C during both expiration and inspiration. Such valves are often marketed as "active exhalation valves", calling attention to their "new" functionality. Nobody seems to remember that simple infant ventilators like the Bourns BP200 were doing pressure controlled ventilation and allowing the patient to breath throughout the ventilatory cycle back in the 1970s.

Figure 3-8. Airway pressure effects with different expiratory pressure devices. A. The water-seal device does not maintain constant pressure and does not allow the patient to inhale, acting like a one-way valve; B. A flow restrictor does not maintain constant pressure but allows limited flow in both directions; C. An electronic demand valve maintains nearly constant pressure and allows unrestricted inspiratory and expiratory flow.

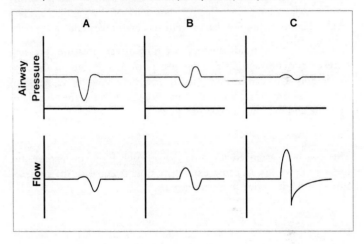

The pressure in the lungs at end expiration (immediately before the start of inspiration) can be higher than the set PEEP. **Dynamic hyperinflation** is the process by which lung volume increases whenever insufficient exhalation time prevents the respiratory system from returning to its resting end-expiratory equilibrium volume between breath cycles. This can occur because the breathing frequency is too high, expiratory resistance is too high, respiratory system compliance is too high, or a combination of the three that make the time constant too long relative to expiratory time (see the discussion about time constants in chapter 4). The term **autoPEEP** is defined as the positive difference between end expiratory alveolar pressure and the end expiratory airway pressure (PEEP or CPAP) selected by the clinician. **Total PEEP** is thus intentionally applied PEEP or CPAP plus autoPEEP.

Mechanical Ventilation

Trapped gas refers to the gas volume associated with dynamic hyperinflation and autoPEEP. Because autoPEEP is the product of trapped gas and respiratory system elastance, the presence of autoPEEP may or may not indicate that the patient's lungs are hyperinflated, depending on elastance or expiratory muscle effort. Also, autoPEEP may be distributed unevenly in the lungs due to variations in regional resistance and elastance.

The most important consequence of excessive autoPEEP is the extra burden on the inspiratory muscles. AutoPEEP is an inspiratory load that must be counterbalanced before inspiratory flow can begin. During assisted ventilation, autoPEEP adds to the triggering pressure, decreasing the effective sensitivity of the ventilator. High levels of autoPEEP may also prevent successful weaning.

AutoPEEP is the residual expiratory flow-driven pressure (pressure = resistance × flow) that remains just prior to the start of the next inspiration. This can be illustrated by again invoking the equation of motion for the respiratory system. For expiration, the ventilator pressure and the muscle pressure are zero:

$$0 = (elastance \times volume) + (resistance \times flow)$$

Extra for Experts

This can be rearranged to show that at each moment in time, the pressure necessary to cause expiratory flow is equal to the pressure stored in the lung due to elastic recoil:

$$-resistance \times flow = elastance \times volume$$

If expiratory flow is interrupted (flow goes to zero), the residual pressure in the lungs equilibrates with the patient circuit and is measured as autoPEEP:

$$autoPEEP = elastance \times residual\ volume$$

If the breathing frequency is high enough to cause autoPEEP, the equation of motion must be modified to account for the extra pressure in the lungs:

$$muscle\ pressure + ventilator\ pressure = (elastance \times volume) + (resistance \times flow) + autoPEEP$$

or equivalently:

$$(muscle\ pressure + ventilator\ pressure) - autoPEEP = (elastance \times volume) + (resistance \times flow)$$

This last form of the equation makes it clear that the sum of muscle pressure and ventilator pressure must be higher than autoPEEP for inspiration to begin. That is, pressure (on the left hand side of the equation) must be greater than zero before volume and flow (on the right hand side) can rise above zero. If a patient is breathing without the assistance of a ventilator, muscle pressure must increase above autoPEEP to start inspiration. Thus, it is obvious that autoPEEP increases the work of breathing.

Review and Consider

21. People sometimes think that CPAP is a form of assisted ventilation. Explain, in terms of the equation of motion, why this is not true.

22. Explain the difference between the terms dynamic hyperinflation, trapped gas, and autoPEEP.

23. Explain the difference between PEEP, autoPEEP and total PEEP.

24. Look at Figure 3-8. Which type of CPAP device imposes the least work of breathing for the patient? How can you tell from the waveforms?

Modes of Ventilation

The objective of mechanical ventilation is to assure that the patient receives the minute ventilation required to satisfy respiratory needs while not damaging the lungs, impairing circulation, or increasing the patient's discomfort. A mode of ventilation is the manner in which a ventilator achieves this objective.

Key Idea

A **mode** is any ventilatory pattern that can be uniquely identified by specifying:

1. the breathing pattern, which includes the primary breath control variable and the breath sequence,

2. the control type, and

3. the specific control strategy.

Note that ventilator manufacturers have dozens of arbitrary names for their modes. Except for a few examples, we will ignore these names for now, preferring to develop a system for understanding and organizing their main characteristics. See Appendix III.

Table 3-1 gives an outline for describing modes of ventilation.[3] This table shows that three basic components of a mode (breathing pattern, control type, and specific control strategy) make up a complete classification for any mode of ventilation.

Table 3-1. Mode classification scheme

I.   **Breathing pattern**
    A. Primary breath control variable
        1. Volume—
        2. Pressure
        3. Dual
    B. Breath sequence
        1. Continuous mandatory ventilation (CMV)
        2. Intermittent mandatory ventilation (IMV)
        3. Continuous spontaneous ventilation (CSV)
II. **Control type**
    A. Set point
    B. Servo
    C. Adaptive
    D. Optimal
III. **Control strategy**
    A. Phase variables (trigger, limit, cycle)
    B. Operational logic (conditional variables, output variables, performance function)

Breathing Pattern

Primary Breath Control Variable

Specifying only the breath control variable for a mode, we can only distinguish among pressure control, volume control, and dual control modes. Often this is all we need to communicate. For example, at the bedside we might simply have to indicate that the

---

[3] Respir Care 2001;46(6):604-621

patient's lung mechanics have become unstable and therefore the mode has been changed from volume control to dual control.

Volume Control

A ventilator can be classified as either a pressure, volume, or flow controller. When classifying modes of ventilation, we do not need to be so specific. Because control of volume implies control of flow and vice versa, we can simply refer to two basic modes of ventilation: volume control and pressure control. Volume control means that tidal volume and inspiratory flow are preset and airway pressure is then dependent upon those settings and respiratory system elastance and resistance (according to the equation of motion).

Pressure Control

Pressure control means that the airway pressure waveform is preset (for example by setting peak inspiratory pressure and end expiratory pressure). Tidal volume and inspiratory flow are then dependent on these settings and the elastance and resistance of the respiratory system.

Dual Control

There are clinical advantages and disadvantages to volume and pressure control, which will be discussed in the clinical application chapter. For now, we can simply say that volume control results in a more stable minute ventilation (and hence more stable blood gases) than pressure control if lung mechanics are unstable. On the other hand, pressure control allows better synchronization with the patient because inspiratory flow is not limited to a preset value.

While it is possible to control only one variable at a time, a ventilator can *automatically* switch between pressure control and volume control in an attempt to guarantee minute ventilation while maximizing patient synchrony. When a ventilator uses both pressure and volume signals to control the breath size, it is called **dual control.**

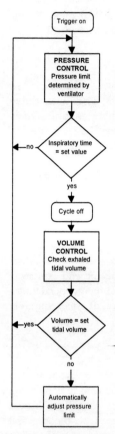

Currently, there are two approaches to dual control. One approach is called **dual control between breaths**. The idea is to control pressure during the breath and to control tidal volume over several breaths through automatic adjustment of the pressure limit. An example of this is the AutoFlow feature on the Dräger Evita 4. Figure 3-9 illustrates the sequence of events. After the breath is triggered on, the control variable is pressure but the inspiratory pressure is limited to a value set by the ventilator, not by the operator (although the operator can set a maximum alarm value the ventilator cannot exceed). Inspiration continues until the set inspiratory time is achieved. Then the ventilator measures the exhaled tidal volume for that breath and compares it to the set value. If the exhaled volume is lower than the set value, the pressure limit for the next breath is automatically increased slightly. If the exhaled volume is higher than the set value, the pressure limit is decreased. In this way, the ventilator controls volume between breaths to compensate for changes in the patient's ventilatory efforts and respiratory system mechanics.

Figure 3-9. Operational logic for dual control between breaths. The cycle variable can be time as shown or flow depending on the specific mode and ventilator.

Another approach to dual control is to switch between pressure control and volume control during a single breath. This is called **dual control within** breaths. One example of this is the Pressure Augment on the Bear 1000. Figure 3-10 illustrates how Pressure Augment works.

Figure 3-10. Operational logic for dual control within breaths as implemented in the Pressure Augment mode on the Bear 1000 ventilator.

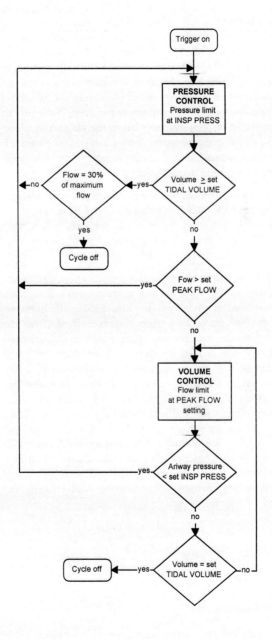

The breath starts out in pressure control while the inspired volume is continually measured and compared to the set tidal volume. If the delivered volume meets the set value, inspiration continues like a Pressure Support[4] breath, cycling off when flow decays to 30% of the initial, maximum value. If, however, the set tidal volume is not met by the time flow decays to the set peak flow value, then the ventilator switches to volume control at a constant inspiratory flow equal to the set peak flow. Inspiration then proceeds until the set tidal volume is met. After the switch to volume control, the ventilator continues to monitor airway pressure. If the patient should make an inspiratory effort late in the inspiratory phase that drops the airway pressure below the set inspiratory pressure limit, the ventilator switches back to pressure control at whatever flow is necessary to meet the patient's demand.

Notice that with Pressure Augment, the breath starts out in pressure control and then switches to volume control (if necessary). It is also possible to start out in volume control and switch to pressure control. This is another form of dual control within breaths. An example is the P_{max} feature on the Dräger Evita 4.

Figure 3-11 is a flow chart for this mode. The breath starts out in volume control with flow limited at the set peak flow value. If the airway pressure stays below the P_{max} setting, then inspiration is cycled off when the set inspiratory time is reached. If the inspiratory time is set longer than the inspiratory flow time (determined by the set tidal volume divided by the set flow) then there will be an inspiratory hold. If the airway pressure reaches the P_{max} setting, the ventilator switches to pressure control and the inspiratory pressure is limited to the P_{max} value. Inspiration then continues until the set inspiratory time is reached and the breath is cycled off. While the breath is in pressure control, if the tidal volume is finally met, inspiratory flow stops and an inspiratory hold ensues until the inspiratory time is met. Otherwise, an alarm is activated. The operator must then assess the patient and make the appropriate ventilator setting changes to balance the tidal volume, inspiratory time, and P_{max} settings.

---

[4] Pressure Support is a mode in which all breaths are patient triggered, pressure limited, and patient cycled.

Figure 3-11. Operational logic for dual control within breaths as implemented using P_{max} on the Dräger Evita 4 ventilator.

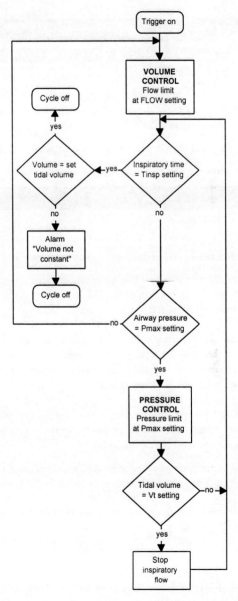

25. What three things must you know to uniquely describe a mode of ventilation?

26. How are the control variables used to classify ventilators different from the breath control variables used to classify modes of ventilation?

27. Explain dual control and its advantages.

28. How do the two types of dual control differ?

Breath Sequence (Mandatory vs. Spontaneous Breaths)

The second component of the breathing pattern specification is the breath sequence. A **breath** is defined as a positive change in airway flow (inspiration) paired with a negative change in airway flow (expiration), both relative to baseline flow and associated with ventilation of the lungs. This definition excludes flow changes caused by hiccups or cardiogenic oscillations. But it allows the superimposition of, say, a spontaneous breath on a mandatory breath or vice versa. For example, the Dräger Eviat 4 allows spontaneous breaths to be superimposed on mandatory breaths in the Airway Pressure Release Ventilation mode. On the other hand, mandatory breaths are superimposed on spontaneous breaths during high frequency oscillatory ventilation.

As noted earlier, not all ventilators will accommodate a spontaneous breath while a mandatory breath is being delivered, which results in greater patient work and discomfort. The longer the mandatory inspiratory time and the more active the patient, the more important this issue becomes.

The classification of modes requires the definition of two basic types of breaths: spontaneous and mandatory. A **spontaneous breath** is a breath for which the patient controls the start time and the tidal volume. That is, the patient both triggers and cycles the breath.

A **mandatory breath** is a breath for which the machine sets the start time and/or the tidal volume. That is, the machine triggers and/or cycles the breath.

Spontaneous breaths may be assisted or unassisted. Some authors define an assisted breath in terms of the phase variables as a breath that is patient triggered and machine cycled. This type of definition only confuses your understanding of modes by adding another name to memorize that is not related to anything else. Besides, it fails in some situations, like expiratory assist (because the definition of assist based on phase variables only addresses inspiration). It even fails for some types of inspiration. For example, when breathing on CPAP, the patient triggers inspiration and the machine could conceivably cycle the breath off (if it thought inspiratory time was too long). Clearly, the ventilator does no work to assist the patient's inspiratory effort, so classifying the breath as "assisted" based on trigger and cycle variables would be misleading.

We have shown above that only two types of breaths need be defined in term of phase variables (mandatory and spontaneous) to classify modes. The wider study of pulmonary mechanics recognizes a more general definition of ventilatory assistance: An **assisted breath** is a breath during which all or part of inspiratory (or expiratory) flow is generated by the ventilator doing work on the patient. In simple terms, if the airway pressure rises above end expiratory pressure during inspiration, the breath is assisted (for example, the Pressure Support mode). It is also possible to assist expiration by dropping airway pressure below end expiratory pressure (such as the Exhalation Assist feature on the Venturi ventilator). If the ventilator generates just enough flow to meet the patient's own demand, then airway pressure will remain at end expiratory level and the breath is not assisted (like CPAP).

Having defined spontaneous and mandatory breaths, there are three possible sequences of breaths, designated as follows:

- *Continuous Mandatory Ventilation (CMV):* all breaths are mandatory

- *Continuous Spontaneous Ventilation (CSV):* all breaths are spontaneous

- *Intermittent Mandatory Ventilation (IMV):* breaths can be either mandatory or spontaneous. Breaths can occur separately or breaths can be superimposed on each other. Spontaneous breaths can be superimposed on mandatory breaths, as in Airway Pressure Release Ventilation (APRV). Alternatively, mandatory breaths can be superimposed on spontaneous breaths, as in high frequency ventilation. When the mandatory breath is patient triggered, it is commonly referred to as **synchronized IMV** (SIMV). However, because the trigger variable can be specified in the description of phase variables, we will use IMV instead of SIMV to designate general breath sequences.

When we add the breath sequence to the control variable in classifying a mode, we get a greater ability to discriminate modes. We can distinguish between, say, pressure controlled IMV and pressure controlled CSV

Key Idea

> Adding the control variable and the breath sequence specifications for a mode gives a very convenient shorthand notation that we can use frequently in everyday clinical practice. It may be all we need to describe the progress of a patient or to compare two different modes.

If we confine ourselves to classifying modes based solely on the breathing pattern, we see that there are only eight possibilities in three groups as shown in Table 3-2. The utility of this system should be immediately obvious. There are dozens of names for modes created by ventilator manufacturers (and sometimes researchers). This makes it easier for marketing people to sell ventilators by making them sound as if they have unique features. However, having many names for the same thing makes it difficult for end users to compare and contrast ventilator capabilities. Table 3-2 allows users to sort all possible modes into just a few categories. This works for modes that have been in use for years as well as new modes and even modes not yet invented. For example, we can identify a new mode, say, Airway Pressure Release Ventilation (APRV), as simply a form of pressure controlled IMV.

See Appendix III for a list of the common ventilator mode names, sorted by ventilator model and matched with their breathing patterns.

Table 3-2. Breathing patterns.

Control Variable	Breath Sequence	Abbreviation
Volume	Continuous Mandatory Ventilation	VC-CMV
	Intermittent Mandatory Ventilation	VC-IMV
Pressure	Continuous Mandatory Ventilation	PC-CMV
	Intermittent Mandatory Ventilation	PC-IMV
	Continuous Spontaneous Ventilation	PC-CSV
Dual	Continuous Mandatory Ventilation	DC-CMV
	Intermittent Mandatory Ventilation	DC-IMV
	Continuous Spontaneous Ventilation	DC-CSV

Review and Consider

29. What is a breath?

30. Why is the distinction between a mandatory and a spontaneous breath a key concept in describing modes?

31. Define the three breath sequences.

32. If there are three breath control variables and three breath sequences, why are there only eight (versus nine) breathing patterns?

33. Give an example of PC-CSV.

34. What is the difference between IMV and SIMV?

35. You know that a patient came out of surgery yesterday and was placed on VC-CMV. Now, two days later, she is on PC-CMV. What might you infer about the patient's progress?

36. If someone told you a patient was placed on "assist control", what would you really know about the mode if you did not know what ventilator was used? What if they said "SIMV"?

37. As an exercise, list all the modes named on a ventilator with which you are familiar. Then sort them into the categories shown in Table 3-2.

38. What breathing pattern does the Pressure Support mode use?

Control Type

We have discussed "control variables" and the differences between pressure, volume, and dual control but, we have not really explained what is meant by "control" in the first place. There are two general ways to control a variable; open loop control and closed loop control.

Open loop control is essentially no control. For example, early high frequency ventilators simply generated pulses of gas flow without measurement or control of pressure, volume, or flow. Flow into the patient was a function of the relative impedances of the respiratory system and the exhalation manifold. Thus, both pressure and volume were affected by any disturbances in the system, such as changing lung mechanics, the patient's ventilatory efforts, and leaks.

Closed loop control is an improvement in that the delivered pressure, volume, and flow can be measured and used as feedback information to control the driving mechanism (like cruise control in an automobile to maintain a constant speed). The actual output is measured (as a feedback signal) and compared to the desired value (intended by the set input). If there is a difference, an error signal is sent to the controller to adjust the output towards the desired output (Figure 3-12.) Thus, inspiratory volumes, flows, and pressures can be made to match or follow specified input values despite disturbances such as changes in patient load and minor leaks in the system. Note that closed loop control does not require an electronic system. A simple pressure regulator is an example of mechanical feedback control.

Figure 3-12. Schematic diagram of a closed loop or feedback control system. The + and – signs indicate that the input setting is compared to the feedback signal and if there is a difference, an error signal is sent to the controller to adjust the output until the difference is zero.

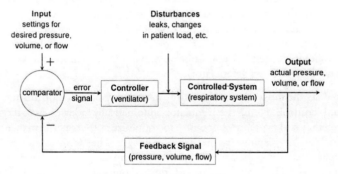

Table 3-1 shows that a more detailed mode description would include the type of control scheme used to manipulate the control variables to produce the permissible breaths. For single variable, closed loop control, setpoint and servo types have been employed. **Setpoint control** means that the output of the ventilator automatically matches a constant, unvarying, operator preset input value (such as the production of a constant inspiratory pressure or flow from breath to breath). **Servo control** means the output automatically follows a dynamic, varying, operator specified input. For example, the Automatic Tube Compensation feature on the Dräger Evita 4 ventilator measures instantaneous flow and forces instantaneous pressure to be equal to flow multiplied by a constant (representing endotracheal tube resistance).

Dual variable, closed loop control (dual control) has used setpoint and adaptive setpoint control. **Setpoint dual control** means that the operator selects both the pressure and volume setpoints (pressure limit and tidal volume) and the ventilator switches between pressure control and volume control as needed. Examples of this are Pressure Limited Ventilation (Dräger Evita 4), Pressure Augment (Bear 1000) and Volume Assured Pressure Support (Bird 8400ST).

Adaptive dual control means that the ventilator automatically adjusts the pressure setpoint (the pressure limit) over several breaths to maintain an operator selected volume setpoint (the target tidal volume) as the mechanics of the respiratory system change. Thus, the ventilator adapts to the need for a changing setpoint. The ventilator typically monitors both exhaled volume and respiratory system compliance on a breath-by-breath basis. Then, if the tidal volume falls below the desired value, the ventilator adjusts the set pressure limit to bring the tidal volume closer to the target (required pressure change = exhaled volume ÷ calculated compliance). We say "target" tidal volume because the ventilator aims to achieve it, but for various reasons, may miss (which should trigger an alarm). Examples of adaptive dual control can be seen in modes like Pressure Regulated Volume Control (Servo 300 ventilator) and Auto Flow (Dräger Evita 4 ventilator).

To date, the most advanced control strategy may be called **optimum dual control**. Here, the ventilator automatically adjusts *both* the pressure and volume setpoints to optimize other performance variables as respiratory mechanics change. The term optimum implies that some measure of system performance is maximized or minimized. The only example of this at present is the Adaptive Support mode on the Hamilton Galileo (perhaps not the best choice of names in light of this classification scheme). In this mode, each breath is pressure controlled and the pressure limit is automatically adjusted between breaths to meet an optimum tidal volume. The optimum tidal volume is based on the estimated minute alveolar ventilation and the optimal frequency. The minute ventilation is estimated from the patient's body weight. The optimal frequency is based on the measured expiratory time constant using an equation that minimizes the work of breathing. The control software also implements "lung protective strategies" by not allowing tidal volume or frequency to get too large or too small. For example, the maximum frequency is based on a minimum inspiratory time equal to one time constant and minimum expiratory time of two time constants.

It is important to recognize that the control types mentioned above represent evolutionary progress in control technology. To visualize this, imagine that we are talking about a computerized law enforcement laser weapon system (sort of a "RoboCop"). At the lowest level of evolution, the system can hit a stationary target (corresponding to setpoint control). The next level up, the system can hit a moving target (servo control). With a little more intelligence, the system can not only hit a moving target, but also preserve the hostage, if you tell it which person is which (adaptive control). At the highest level, the system can identify the target and the hostage on its own (optimal control). Of course, ventilator control technology is not as sophisticated as this, but you get the idea.

Table 3-3 gives a brief summary of the various control types with some examples. This table may seem a bit difficult to comprehend at first. However, you must master it if you really want to know how ventilators work and be able to distinguish the true capabilities of one model of ventilator from another. This is particularly important if you are in a position either to purchase (or sell) ventilators or to train people on how to use them. In these cases you need to compare different types of ventilators and modes of ventilation. You will not find this type of information in the ventilator manufacturer's literature. In fact, you will know that you have understood when you can look at the description of a mode in any ventilator operator's manual and recognize what control type it uses.

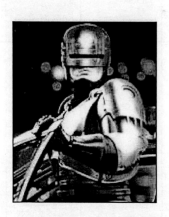

Table 3-3. Control types, descriptions, and examples.

Control Type	Description	Example Control Scheme	Example Mode	Example Ventilator
Setpoint	Output matches fixed input	Tidal volume or peak pressure held constant by adjusting control variable	Pressure Control Assist Control Pressure Support	Siemens Servo Hamilton Galileo PB 840
Servo	Output matches dynamic input	Pressure made proportional to volume and/or flow	Proportional Assist Automatic Tube Compensation	Not available in US Dräger Evita 4
Setpoint Dual Control	Automatic switch between pressure and volume control to maintain operator defined setpoints	Volume control overrides pressure control within breath if set tidal volume not met	Pressure Limited Ventilation Volume Assured Pressure Support	Dräger Evita 4 Bird 8400ST
Adaptive Dual Control	Automatic adjustment of pressure setpoint to maintain an operator selected volume setpoint	Pressure limit adjusted to maintain set tidal volume, using lung mechanics	Pressure Regulated Volume Control AutoFlow	Siemens Servo 300 Drager Evita 4
Optimal Dual Control	Automatic adjustment of both pressure and volume setpoints to minimize or maximize other variables	Pressure limit and tidal volume adjusted to minimize work of breathing, using lung mechanics	Adaptive Support Ventilation	Hamilton Galileo

- 56 -

39. Explain the difference between open loop control and closed loop control.

40. This section describes five different control types. They appeared on commercial ventilators at different times and may be considered to have followed an evolutionary progression. Name the control strategies and put them in order from the simplest to the most advanced.

41. Earlier we said that there were two types of dual control, one that acted within breaths and one that acted between breaths. Relate these two types to the control schemes described in this section.

42. What do you think are the motives for continually developing more sophisticated types of ventilator control?

Control Strategy

Phase Variables

So far, we have shown how modes of ventilation can be described at various levels of detail, depending on how and with whom we need to communicate. At the highest level of detail, we can fully characterize a mode by adding the specific control strategy it employs. This begins with naming the phase variables (pressure, volume, flow, and time), followed by detailing the operational logic, and, if necessary, giving the parameter values used in the conditional statements.

As we have seen, a mode is a pattern of mandatory and spontaneous breaths. Because these breaths may vary drastically in the way they are controlled, we must specify the phase variables for both types of breaths. For example, a ventilator may provide volume controlled mandatory breaths that are time triggered, flow limited, and volume cycled, interspersed with pressure controlled spontaneous breaths that are pressure triggered, pressure limited, and flow cycled. Each type of breath has a completely different set of phase variables.

Operational Logic

Ventilators can also use pressure, volume, flow, or time (and their derivatives such as minute ventilation) as conditional variables. A **conditional variable** is used by a ventilator's operational logic system to make decisions. The **operational logic** of a ventilator is a simple description of how the computer uses the conditional variables. Operational logic often takes the form of "if-then" statements. That is, *if* the value of a conditional variable reaches some preset level, *then* some action occurs to change the ventilatory pattern.

For example, *if* a preset time interval has elapsed (the sigh interval), *then* the ventilator switches to the sigh pattern. Another example is the switch between patient-triggered breaths and machine-triggered breaths that occur during intermittent mandatory ventilation. An even more sophisticated example is illustrated in Figure 3-10 showing the operational logic for dual control within breaths.

The Complete Specification

A complete classification for any mode of ventilation is the specification of :

Key Idea

> 1. the breathing pattern that the mode can produce (breath control variable and breath sequence),
>
> 2. the type of control (setpoint, servo, adaptive, or optimal control),
>
> 3. the specific control strategy (phase variables, conditional variables and, operational logic) it uses, for both mandatory and spontaneous breaths.

A complete description helps us to distinguish between different modes that look the same on graphics monitors and suggests what the operator must do to set the controls. For example, Pressure Support (any ventilator) is PC-CSV for which the operator sets the sensitivity (trigger variable) and pressure limit (limit variable). In contrast, Volume Assist (Siemens 300) is DC-CSV which looks similar to Pressure Support on a graphics monitor but the operator must set a tidal volume (conditional variable) in addition to sensitivity and pressure limit.

Specifying the phase variables and operational logic also helps to distinguish between modes with similar sounding names. For example, on the Bear 1000, "Assist Control" is VC-CMV but "Assist Control + Pressure Augment" is DC-IMV, about as different as two modes can get. In a similar manner, specifying the phase variables and operational logic helps to distinguish among the four types of DC-IMV on the Dräger Evita 4.

Table 3-4 shows how both simple and complex modes of ventilation can be completely described. Notice that the names of the modes, themselves, give you very little idea of how they work. A name like "Bi-Level" (on the Puritan Bennett 840 ventilator) is practically meaningless, even if you know it is a form of pressure control. All pressure control modes use two ("bi") levels of pressure. However, the name does serve to remind us that this particular form of PC-IMV is different from, say, that offered by the Bear Cub ventilator. The Cub does not have any trigger or cycle variables for spontaneous breaths, meaning it cannot recognize and react to the patient's breathing efforts. All it can do is provide a pressure limit. In contrast, the PB 840 does recognize and respond to spontaneous breaths using pressure or flow triggering and flow cycling. Thus, it exhibits the "active exhalation manifold" feature discussed previously (see Figure 3-8).

If we look at the operational logic of the three ventilators shown in Table 3-4, it becomes obvious that there is a progression of complexity. The Bear Cub has no operational logic; its control circuit is little more than an automatic on/off switch. The Bi-Level mode on the PB 840 uses simple control logic to switch between two different sets of phase variables, one for mandatory breaths and one for spontaneous breaths. The Mandatory Minute Ventilation mode on the Evita 4 is the most complex. It uses two conditional variables, minute ventilation and tidal volume, to implement dual control and to maintain a level of support while responding to the patient's ventilatory demand.

It is instructive to compare modes as shown in Table 3-4 not only to appreciate their relative complexity but to understand what input variables the operator must consider. On the Cub, you only set pressure, frequency, and I:E ratio. On the Evita 4, you must set pressure, frequency, volume, flow, and minute ventilation.

Table 3-4. Examples of how to describe simple, moderately complex and complex modes using the classification scheme shown in Table 3-1.

Ventilator Name	Bear Cub	PB 840	Dräger Evita 4
Mode Name	CMV/IMV	Bi-Level	MMV + autoflow
1. Breathing Pattern	PC-IMV	PC-IMV	DC-IMV
2. Control Type	set point	set point	adaptive
3. Control Strategy			
Mandatory Phase Variables			
Trigger	time	time	time
Limit	pressure	pressure	volume, flow
Cycle	time	time	volume
Spontaneous Phase Variables			
Trigger	none	pressure, flow	flow
Limit	pressure	pressure	pressure
Cycle	none	flow	time
Conditional variables	none	none	minute ventilation tidal volume
Operational Logic	none	switch between mandatory and spontaneous breaths	if set minute ventilation is not achieved by spontaneous breaths, trigger mandatory breaths; if set tidal volume not achieved, then adjust pressure limit

43. Why do we need to include the phase variables in a description of a mode?

44. What is meant by the operational logic of a mode?

45. The mode called CMV/IMV on the Bear Cub is a form of PC-IMV. So is the BiLevel mode on the PB 840. They look similar on a graphics monitor. How can we distinguish between them? (*Hint: examine Table 3-4.*)

46. Pick a mode you are familiar with and classify it using the format in Table 3-4.

Alarm Systems

The ventilator classification scheme described previously centers on the basic functions of input, control, and output. If any of these functions fails, a life-threatening situation may result. Thus, ventilators are equipped with various types of alarms, which may be classified in the same manner as the other major ventilator characteristics.

The goal of ventilator alarms is to warn of events. An "alarm event" is any condition or occurrence that requires clinician awareness or action. Technical events are those involving an inadvertent change in the ventilator's performance; patient events are those involving a change in the patient's clinical status that can be detected by the ventilator. A ventilator may be equipped with any conceivable vital sign monitor, but we will limit the scope here to include the ventilator's mechanical/electronic operation and those variables associated with the mechanics of breathing (pressure, volume, flow, and time).

Alarms may be audible, visual, or both, depending on the seriousness of the alarm condition. Visual alarms may be as simple as colored lights or may be as complex as alphanumeric messages to the operator indicating the exact nature of the fault condition. Specifications for an alarm event should include (1) conditions that trigger the alarm, (2) the alarm response in the form of audible and/or visual messages, (3) any associated ventilator response such as termination of inspiration or failure to operate, and (4) whether the alarm must be manually reset or resets itself when the alarm condition is rectified. Table 3-5 outlines the various levels of alarm priority along with alarm characteristics and appropriate alarm categories. Alarm categories are based on the ventilator classification scheme and are detailed below.

Not all ventilators have all the alarms listed in Table 3-5, of course, and a particular manufacturer may not treat the alarm event with the exact priority listed. However, the table provides a way to think about the relative importance of alarms and alerts. For example, the table shows that an alarm for a critical malfunction should be mandatory, redundant, non-canceling, both audible and visual. In comparison, a non-critical malfunction alarm does not need to be redundant and non-canceling.

Note that the events in Table 3-5 can be divided into two groups; those that relate to ventilator function and those that indicate patient condition. The list of events for patient status could be greatly expanded. This is because the ventilator can monitor a variety of calculated parameters (such as patient resistance and compliance) and because the ventilator can be interfaced with other devices including saturation and end tidal carbon dioxide monitors.

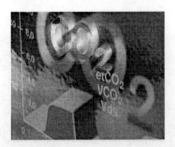 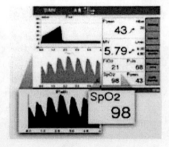

Table 3-5. Classification of Desirable Ventilator Alarms

	Event Priority			
	Level 1 Critical malfunction	Level 2 Non-critical malfunction	Level 3 Pt. status change	Level 4 Operator alert
Alarm Characteristics				
Mandatory	yes	yes	no	yes
Redundant	yes	no	no	no
Noncancelling	yes	no	no	yes
Audible	yes	yes	yes	no
Visual	yes	yes	yes	yes
Automatic backup	yes	no	no	no
Automatic Reset				
Audible	yes	yes	yes	yes
Visual	no	yes	yes	yes
Alarm Events				
Input				
Electrical power	yes	n/a	n/a	n/a
Pneumatic power	yes	n/a	n/a	n/a
Control Circuit				
Inverse I:E ratio	no	yes	no	yes
Incompatible settings	no	no	no	yes
Mech./elect. fault	yes	no	no	no
Output				
Pressure	yes	yes	yes	yes
Volume	yes	yes	yes	yes
Flow	yes	yes	yes	yes
Minute ventilation	yes	yes	yes	yes
Time	yes	yes	yes	yes
Insp. gas (FiO_2/temp.)	yes	yes	no	yes

Critical = immediately life threatening
Non-critical = not immediately life threatening
Patient status = neurologic ventilatory drive, mechanics, hemodynamics, etc.
Operator alert = warning of potentially dangerous settings.
Redundant = alarm mechanism designed in duplicate or backed up by related mechanisms
Non-canceling = operator cannot reset alarm until the alarm condition has been corrected
Automatic reset = alarm automatically cancelled when alarm condition has been corrected
n/a = not applicable

Mechanical Ventilation

Ventilator alarms have recently taken on new importance. The Joint Committee for Accreditation of Health Care Organizations (JCAHO) released a sentinel event report in January 2002 involving ventilators. A sentinel event is any unexpected occurrence that results in death or serious permanent injury. The JCAHO report described 23 ventilator events that resulted in 19 deaths and 4 comas. Sixty five percent of the events were related to the malfunction or misuse of a ventilator alarm. Fifty two percent were related to tubing disconnection and 26% were related to a dislodged airway. A "root cause" analysis revealed that fully 87% of the events were due to inadequate orientation of the staff. In 79% of the cases where equipment failure was the cause, alarms were either not set or not checked to make sure they could be heard. These are shocking statistics that indicate the need for understanding ventilator alarms.

Input Power Alarms

Loss of Electric Power

Most ventilators have some sort of battery backup in the case of electrical power failure, even if the batteries only power alarms. Ventilators typically have alarms that are activated if the electrical power is cut off while the machine is still switched on (e.g. if the power cord is accidentally pulled out of the wall socket). If the ventilator is designed to operate on battery power (like transport ventilators), there is usually an alarm to warn of a low-battery condition.

Loss of Pneumatic Power

Ventilators that use pneumatic power have alarms that are activated if either the oxygen or air supply is cut off or reduced below some specified driving pressure. In most cases, the alarm is activated by an electronic pressure switch but sometimes the alarm is pneumatically operated as a part of the blender (e.g., Siemens Servo 900C).

Control Circuit Alarms

Control circuit alarms are those that either warn the operator that the set control variable parameters are incompatible (perhaps an inverse I:E ratio setting) or indicate that some aspect of a ventilator self-test has failed. In the latter case, there may be something wrong with the ventilator control circuitry itself (like a microprocessor failure) and the ventilator generally responds with some generic message like "Ventilator Inoperative".

Output Alarms

Output alarms are those that are triggered by an unacceptable state of the ventilator's output. More specifically, an output alarm is activated when the value of a control variable (pressure, volume, flow, or time) falls outside an expected range. Some possibilities include the following:

Pressure

High and Low Airway Pressure

High alarms occur for such things as endotracheal tube obstruction, when the patient coughs or if the inspiratory flow is increased during volume controlled ventilation. Low alarms occur if the patient becomes disconnected from the ventilator or a leak develops in the patient circuit.

High and Low Mean Airway Pressure

These alarms indicate a possible leak in the patient circuit or a change in ventilatory pattern that might lead to a change in the patient's oxygenation status (within reasonable limits, oxygenation is roughly proportional to mean airway pressure).

High and Low Baseline Pressure

These alarms indicate a possible patient circuit or exhalation manifold obstruction (or inadvertent PEEP) and disconnection of the patient from the patient circuit, respectively.

Failure to Return to Baseline

Failure of airway pressure to return to baseline within a specified period indicates a possible patient circuit obstruction or exhalation manifold malfunction.

Volume

High and Low Exhaled Volume

These alarms indicate changes in respiratory system time constant or patient effort during pressure-controlled ventilation, leaks around the endotracheal tube or from the lungs, or possible disconnection of the patient from the patient circuit.

Flow

High and Low Expired Minute Volume

These alarms indicate hyperventilation (or possible machine self-triggering) and possible apnea or disconnection of the patient from the patient circuit, respectively.

Time

High and Low Ventilatory Frequency

When these alarms occur, hyperventilation (or possible machine self-triggering) and possible apnea, respectively, may be happening.

Inappropriate Inspiratory Time

An "inspiratory time too long" alarm indicates a possible patient circuit obstruction or exhalation manifold malfunction. An "inspiratory time too short" alarm indicates that adequate tidal volume may not be delivered (in a pressure-controlled mode) or that gas distribution in the lungs may not be optimal.

Inappropriate Expiratory Time

An "expiratory time too long" alarm may indicate apnea. An "expiratory time too short" alarm may warn of alveolar gas trapping (expiratory time should be greater than or equal to five time constants of the respiratory system).

Inspired Gas

Inspired gas conditions have been standard alarm parameters for some time. These include High/low inspired gas temperature and High/low inspired oxygen concentration.

Self Assessment Questions

Definitions

- Transrespiratory system pressure

- Transairway pressure

- Transthoracic pressure

- Transpulmonary pressure

- Transalveolar pressure

- Transmural pressure

- Elastance

- Compliance

- Resistance

- Total ventilatory support

- Partial ventilatory support

- Series connection

- Parallel connection

- Control variable

- Phase variable

- Limit variable

- Cycle variable

- Trigger

- Sensitivity

- Limit

- Cycle

- Expiratory time

- Expiratory flow time

- Expiratory **pause time**

- Inspiratory time

- Inspiratory flow time

- Inspiratory **pause time**

- Total cycle time

- Ventilatory period

- Dynamic hyperinflation

- Trapped gas

- PEEP

- AutoPEEP

- Total PEEP

- Mode (of ventilation)

- Volume control

- Pressure control

- Dual control

- Dual control between breaths

- Dual control within breaths

- Breath

- Spontaneous breath

- Mandatory breath

- Assisted breath

- CMV

- IMV

- CSV

- Pressure Support

- Synchronized IMV

- Closed loop (feedback) control

- Setpoint control

- Servo control

- Setpoint dual control

- Adaptive dual control

- Optimum control

- Conditional variable

- Operational logic

True or False

1. In the equation of motion, pressure, volume and flow are variables while elastance and resistance are constants.

2. The pressure driving inspiration is transthoracic pressure.

3. The pressure you read on a ventilator's airway pressure monitor is actually transrespiratory system pressure.

4. When two compliances are connected in series, the total compliance of the system is greater than the compliance of either one of the two components.

5. An example of two compliances connected in series is the compliance of the lungs in combination with the compliance of the chest wall.

6. A parallel connection of resistances has a lower resistance than neither component.

7. Compliances in parallel add like resistances in series.

8. If the ventilator controls pressure, the pressure waveform will remain constant with changes in respiratory system mechanics but volume and flow will vary.

9. If the ventilator controls volume or flow, the volume and flow waveforms will remain constant with changes in respiratory system mechanics but pressure will vary.

10. What distinguishes a volume controller from a flow controller is that a volume controller actually measures the delivered volume and uses the signal to control the ventilator output.

11. An inspiratory hold can only occur if the inspiratory time is shorter than the inspiratory flow time.

12. Theoretically, flow triggering imposes less work on the patient than pressure triggering.

13. Inspiration ends when airway pressure exceeds the set pressure limit.

14. A breath that is volume limited will normally be time cycled.

15. If the ventilatory period is decreased, the ventilatory frequency has to increase.

16. If the I:E ratio is changed, the frequency must also change.

17. Increasing the I:E ratio too much can result in dynamic hyperinflation.

18. The most important consequence of excessive autoPEEP is the extra burden on the inspiratory muscles.

19. The equation of motion shows that a ventilator can control up to three variables at the same time.

20. Volume control generally results in more stable minute ventilation than pressure control, but pressure control allows better synchronization with the patient.

21. Dual control is an attempt to obtain the gas exchange stability of volume control while maximizing patient synchronization.

22. Dual control between breaths requires more operator preset variables than dual control within breaths.

23. CPAP is a form of assisted breath.

24. The proof that the patient's breathing effort is assisted by the ventilator is that the airway pressure rises above

baseline during inspiration or falls below baseline during expiration.

25. CPAP is a form of CSV.

26. In open loop control, feedback signals are compared to the input signals. If there is a difference, an error signal is sent to the controller to adjust the output until the difference is zero.

27. Setpoint dual control is a more sophisticated control strategy than optimum control.

28. Proportional Assist is an example of servo control.

29. A particular mode of ventilation may have a completely different set of phase variables for mandatory and spontaneous breaths.

30. Minute ventilation is a conditional variable for the Mandatory Minute Ventilation mode.

31. To completely describe a mode you need to specify the breathing pattern, the control type and the control strategy for mandatory breaths only.

Multiple Choice

1. The four basic mechanical characteristics of a ventilator are:

    a. Input power, power conversion, control system, output

    b. Pressure, volume, flow, time

    c. Breathing pattern, control type, phase variables, operational logic

    d. Volume control, pressure control, mandatory breaths, spontaneous breaths

2. All of the following are true about the equation of motion for the respiratory system except:

    a. Equates muscle pressure and ventilator pressure to elastic and resistive loads.

    b. Relates pressure, volume and flow as functions of time.

    c.   Treats volume, pressure, and flow as constants while elastance and resistance are variables.

    d.   Is a mathematical model describing the physical characteristics of a flow conducting tube connected to an elastic compartment.

3.   Compliance is defined as:

    a. Δvolume/Δpressure

    b. Δpressure/Δvolume

    c. Δflow/Δpressure

    d. Δpressure/Δflow

4.   Resistance is defined as:

    a. Δvolume/Δpressure

    b. Δpressure/Δvolume

    c. Δflow/Δpressure

    d. Δpressure/Δflow

5.   Elastance is defined as:

    a. Δvolume/Δpressure

    b. Δpressure/Δvolume

    c. Δflow/Δpressure

    d. Δpressure/Δflow

6.   Which of the following components of the patient-ventilator system are connected in series:

    a.   Left and right lungs

    b.   Patient circuit compliance and respiratory system compliance

    c.   Endotracheal tube resistance and airways resistance

    d.   None of the above

7.   Which of the following components of the respiratory system are connected in parallel:

    a.   Lung compliance and chest wall compliance

    b.   Left and right mainstem bronchi

    c.   Endotracheal tube resistance and airways resistance

    d.   None of the above

8.   The compliance of the lungs is 0.2 L/cm H_2O and that of the chest wall is also 0.2 L/cm H_2O. What is the total compliance of the respiratory system?

    a.   0.4 L/cm H_2O

    b.   0.2 L/cm H_2O

    c.   0.1 L/cm H_2O

    d.   not enough information to perform calculation

9.   The resistance of the endotracheal tube is 10 cm $H_2O/L/s$ and the resistance of the respiratory system is 5.0 cm $H_2O/L/s$. What is the total resistance of the intubated patient?

    a.   5 cm $H_2O/L/s$

    b.   15 cm $H_2O/L/s$

    c.   3.3 cm $H_2O/L/s$

    d.   not enough information to perform calculation

10.   A ventilator is connected to a lung simulator and a particular mode is selected. As the resistance and compliance of the simulator is changed, you notice that the tidal volume remains constant but airway pressure changes. You conclude the following that the ventilator is a:

    a.   Pressure controller

    b.   Time controller

    c.   Flow controller

    d.   None of the above

11.   A ventilator is connected to a lung simulator and a particular mode is selected. As the resistance and compliance of the simulator is changed, you notice that the airway pressure remains constant but the tidal volume changes. You conclude the following that the ventilator is a:

   a.   Pressure controller

   b.   Time controller

   c.   Flow controller

   d.   None of the above

12. The trigger variable

   a.   Starts inspiration

   b.   Determines peak pressure or flow during inspiration

   c.   Starts expiration

   d.   Determines baseline pressure

13. The limit variable

   a.   Starts inspiration

   b.   Determines peak pressure, volume, or flow during inspiration

   c.   Starts expiration

   d.   Determines baseline pressure

14. The cycle variable

   a.   Starts inspiration

   b.   Determines peak pressure or flow during inspiration

   c.   Starts expiration

   d.   Determines baseline pressure

15. If the flow trigger threshold is changed from 1.0 L/min to 2.0 L/min

   a.   The sensitivity is decreased

   b.   The sensitivity is increased

   c.   The ventilator may auto-trigger

   d.   The frequency will be greater

16. If a ventilator that is a flow controller and the operator increases the inspiratory time so that it is longer than the inspiratory flow time, then

   a.   The ventilator will be time cycled

b. The ventilator will be volume limited

c. The I:E ratio will be larger

d. All of the above

17. If the inspiratory time is 1 second and the expiratory time is 3 seconds, all of the following are true except:

a. The I:E ratio is 1:3

b. The I:E ratio is 1:4

c. The frequency is 15 breaths/min

d. The duty cycle is 25%

18. Examine Figure 3-8. Which CPAP system do you think would impose the least work of breathing on the patient?

a. A

b. B

c. C

d. They are all the same because they are all CPAP devices

19. Dynamic hyperinflation might be caused by any of the following except:

a. Increased airway resistance

b. Increased ventilatory frequency

c. Decreased lung elastance

d. Increased expiratory time

20. All of the following are true about autoPEEP except:

a. It places an extra burden on the inspiratory muscles.

b. It adds to the triggering pressure, decreasing the effective sensitivity of the ventilator.

c. It may prevent successful weaning.

d. It can be avoided by increasing the inspiratory time.

21. A mode can be uniquely identified by specifying all but which of the following:

    a.   The breathing pattern

    b.   The control type.

    c.   The specific control strategy.

    d.   The name the ventilator manufacturer uses to describe it.

22. When a ventilator automatically switches between pressure control and volume control for mandatory breaths it is referred to as:

    a.   SIMV+Pressure support

    b.   Dual control

    c.   Volume targeted ventilation

    d.   Proportional Assist ventilation

23. Examine Figure 3-9. It says that:

    a.   Inspiration starts in volume control and switches to pressure control before inspiration ends.

    b.   Inspiration ends when the set tidal volume is met.

    c.   The pressure limit is adjusted if the tidal volume is not met.

    d.   The pressure limit is adjusted after every breath.

24. Examine Figure 3-10. It says that:

    a.   The breath is cycled off as soon as the set tidal volume is met.

    b.   Pressure control switches to volume control if the tidal volume is not met and inspiratory flow equals the set peak flow.

    c.   Volume control switches to pressure control when the tidal volume is met.

    d.   Once pressure control switches to volume control, it can never go back to pressure control.

25. Examine Figure 3-11. It says that:

    a.   The breath is cycled off as soon as the set tidal volume is met.

b. Pressure control switches to volume control if the tidal volume is not met and inspiratory flow equals the set peak flow. ⎯

c. Volume control switches to pressure control when the P_{max} setting is met.

d. Pressure control switches to volume control when the set inspiratory time is met.

26. All of the following are mandatory breaths except one that is:

   a. Machine triggered and machine cycled

   b. Patient triggered and machine cycled

   c. Machine triggered and patient cycled

   d. Patient triggered and patient cycled

27. An assisted breath is one for which:

   a. The patient triggers inspiratory flow from the ventilator.

   b. Inspiration is patient triggered and machine cycled.

   c. The patient breathes on CPAP.

   d. All or part of inspiratory (or expiratory) flow is generated by the ventilator doing work on the patient.

28. The breath sequence in which most breaths are patient triggered and machine cycled but there is an occasional machine triggered, machine cycled breath is called:

   a. Continuous mandatory ventilation (CMV)

   b. Intermittent mandatory ventilation (IMV)

   c. Synchronized intermittent mandatory ventilation (SIMV)

   d. Continuous spontaneous ventilation (CSV)

29. Why does adding the control variable to the breath sequence make the mode classification more useful?

   a. It helps to distinguish between pressure and volume control modes that have entirely different effects on the patient.

    b.   It helps to group together many modes with different brand names.

    c.   It sorts dozens of specific modes into just eight categories, simplifying learning.

    d.   All of the above.

30. Controlling a high frequency ventilator's frequency and duty cycle only, letting pressure and flow be dependent on lung mechanics, is an example of:

    a.   Open loop control

    b.   Closed loop control

    c.   Dual control

    d.   Adaptive control

31. Using _____ control, the ventilator switches automatically between volume control and pressure control:

    a.   Open loop control

    b.   Servo control

    c.   Dual control

    d.   Setpoint control

32. A mode of ventilation in which all breaths are machine triggered, pressure limited to the same value and machine cycled uses:

    a.   Setpoint control

    b.   Servo control

    c.   Adaptive control

    d.   Optimal control

33. Automatic Tube Compensation is a mode that adjusts the inspiratory pressure in proportion to the patient's inspiratory flow demand. This is an example of:

    a.   Setpoint control

    b.   Servo control

    c.   Adaptive control

    d.   Optimal control

34. During Pressure Limited Ventilation on the Drager Evita 4 ventilator, the breath starts out in pressure control but then switches to volume control. This is an example of:

    a.   Servo control

    b.   Setpoint dual control

    c.   Adaptive dual control

    d.   Optimal control

35. Pressure Regulated Volume Control on the Servo ventilator adjusts the pressure limit from breath to breath, depending on respiratory system mechanics, to assure a fixed tidal volume is delivered. This is an example of:

    a.   Servo control

    b.   Setpoint dual control

    c.   Adaptive dual control

    d.   Optimal control

36. The Hamilton Galileo has a mode that adjusts the pressure limit from breath to breath to assure the patient receives a variable tidal volume that is appropriate for his weight and respiratory system mechanics. This is an example of:

    a.   Servo control

    b.   Setpoint dual control

    c.   Adaptive dual control

    d.   Optimal control

37. Adding the phase variables to the mode classification description allows us to:

    a.   Distinguish between mandatory and spontaneous breaths.

    b.   Tell how the ventilator switches between volume and pressure control.

    c.   Define the feedback control system.

    d.   Just get more confused.

38. The operational logic of a ventilator is:

    a. A description of how the computer uses the conditional variables.

    b. Describes how the ventilator switches between phase variables with "if-then" statements.

    c. Tells how the ventilator switches between mandatory and spontaneous breaths.

    d. All of the above.

39. A complete specification or description of a mode consists of the:

    a. Ventilator name, mode name, and breathing pattern.

    b. Mode name, breathing pattern, and operational logic.

    c. Control strategy, breathing pattern, and phase variables.

    d. Breathing pattern, control type, and control strategy.

Key Ideas

1. Write the equation of motion for the respiratory system.

2. When a patient is connected to a ventilator, how can you tell by looking at the pressure waveform if a particular breath is assisted or unassisted?

3. What are the four variables in the equation of motion that a ventilator can control?

4. Name the four phase variables.

5. Write an equation relating expiratory time, expiratory flow time and expiratory pause time.

6. What is the difference between a volume limited and a volume cycled breath?

7. Write an equation relating inspiratory time, inspiratory flow time, and inspiratory pause time.

8. Write an equation relating total cycle time, inspiratory time, and expiratory time.

9. What happens if inspiratory time is longer than inspiratory flow time? How would you recognize this on a ventilator graphics display?

10. A mode can be uniquely specified by what three characteristics?

11. In the Pressure Support mode, the patient can trigger each breath. The breath cycles off when inspiratory flow decreases to some preset threshold. Inspiratory flow decreases either because the patient's lungs are full (passive inspiration) or because the patient actively tries to exhale. Would you consider breaths in this mode to be mandatory or spontaneous? Why?

12. Why is it not enough to say that a patient is on IMV?

"The full advantage of the newly available ventilator modes and features will be realized only if your facility is willing and able to dedicate time to an extensive in-house training program Often, clinicians overlook the new, and perhaps more optimal, modes because they are more familiar with the older modes."

ECRI Health Devices July 2002, Volume 31, Number 7

4. HOW TO USE MODES OF VENTILATION

The clinical use of the many available modes of ventilation is a much debated topic. A full coverage of all the issues is beyond the scope of this presentation. However, we will review the clinical application of the major breathing patterns shown in Table 3-2. This should provide the student with a solid understanding of the basic approaches to ventilatory support and a framework for learning more through actual experience and further reading.

Volume Control vs. Pressure Control

Figure 4-1 illustrates the important variables for *volume control* modes. It shows that the primary variable we wish to control is the patient's minute ventilation. Minute ventilation is usually adjusted by means of a set tidal volume and frequency (rate), but some ventilators require you to set minute volume directly. In addition, some ventilators allow you to set rate directly while on others rate is an indirect result of the inspiratory and expiratory time settings. Tidal volume is a function of the set inspiratory flow and the set inspiratory time. Inspiratory time is affected by the set frequency and, if adjustable, the set I:E ratio. The mathematical relations among all these variables are given in Table 4-1.

With *pressure control* modes, the goal is again to maintain adequate minute ventilation. However, when pressure is controlled, tidal volume and thus minute ventilation are dependent not only on the ventilator's pressure settings but also on the elastance and resistance of the patient's respiratory system. This makes minute ventilation and gas exchange less stable in pressure control modes than volume control modes. Figure 4-2 shows the important variables for pressure control modes.

Figure 4-1. Influence diagram showing the relations among the key variables during volume controlled mechanical ventilation.

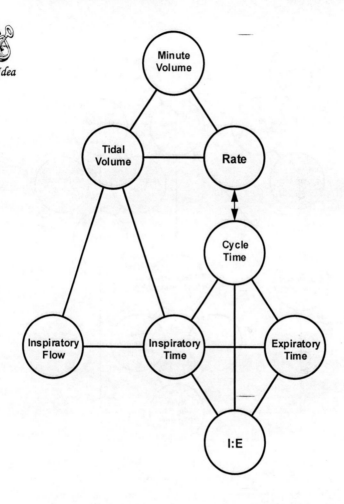

Key Idea

This diagram represents the most fundamental ideas of mechanical ventilation. Without a complete understanding of the variables and how they are related, you will not be able to understand how to manage even the simplest mode of ventilation.

Figure 4-2. Influence diagram showing the relations among the key variables during pressure controlled mechanical ventilation. The shaded circles show variables that are not set on the ventilator.

Key Idea

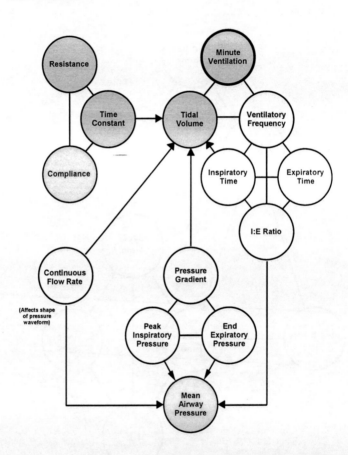

This figure shows that tidal volume is the result of the pressure gradient (peak inspiratory pressure minus end expiratory pressure) and the patient's lung mechanics as well as the inspiratory time. On some ventilators, the **pressure rise time** (the speed with which the peak inspiratory pressure is achieved, sometimes called pressure slope or flow acceleration) is adjustable. That adjustment affects the shape of the pressure waveform and thus the peak inspiratory pressure, the tidal volume, and the mean airway pressure. As the mean airway pressure rises (within reasonable limits), arterial oxygen tension rises. Mean airway pressure is proportional to the area under the pressure-time curve, so any change of ventilator settings that increases the area (such as increasing the inspiratory or expiratory pressure limit, the flow, or the I:E ratio). ___

Figure 4-3 shows the Radford nomogram, used for determining appropriate volume control settings for different sized patients from infants to adults.

Figure 4-3. Radford nomogram for determining appropriate settings for volume controlled ventilation of patients with normal lungs. Patients with paremchymal lung disease should be ventilated with tidal volumes no larger than 6 mL/kg.

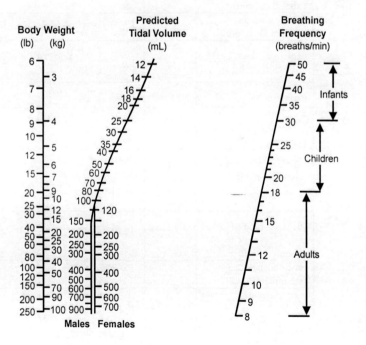

Table 4-1. Equations relating the variables are shown in Figures 4-1 and 4-3.

Mode	Parameter	Symbol	Equation
volume control	tidal volume (L)	V_T	$V_T = \dot{V}_E \div f = \overline{\dot{V}_I} \times T_I$
	mean inspiratory flow (L/min)	$\overline{\dot{V}_I}$	$\overline{\dot{V}_I} = 60 \times V_T \div T_I$
pressure control	tidal volume (L)	V_T	$V_T = \Delta P \times C \times \left(1 - e^{-t/\tau}\right)$
	inspiratory flow (L/s)	$\dot{V}_I$	$\dot{V}_I = \left(\dfrac{\Delta P}{R}\right)\left(e^{-t/\tau}\right)$
both modes	pressure gradient (cmH$_2$O)	ΔP	$\Delta P = PIP - PEEP$
	minute ventilation exhaled (L/min)	$\dot{V}_E$	$\dot{V}_E = f \times V_T$
	minute alveolar ventilation (L/min)	$\dot{V}_A$	$\dot{V}_A = f \times (V_T - V_D)$
	expiratory flow (L/s)	$\dot{V}_E$	$\dot{V}_E = -\left(\dfrac{\Delta P}{R}\right)\left(e^{-t/\tau}\right)$
	expiratory volume (L)	V	$V = C\Delta P\left(e^{-t/RC}\right)$
	total cycle time or ventilatory period (seconds)	TCT	$TCT = T_I + T_E = 60 \div f$
	ventilatory frequency (cycles/minute)	f	$f = 60 \div (T_I + T_E)$ $f = \left(\dfrac{60}{I}\right)\left(\dfrac{I}{I + E}\right)$
	I:E ratio; ratio of inspiratory time to expiratory time	$I{:}E$	$I : E = T_I : T_E = \dfrac{T_I}{T_E}$
	time constant (seconds)	τ	$\tau = R \times C$
	resistance (cmH$_2$O/L/s) compliance (L/cmH$_2$O	R C	$R = \dfrac{\Delta P}{\Delta \dot{V}}$ $\qquad$ $C = \dfrac{\Delta V}{\Delta P}$
	elastance (cmH$_2$O/L)	E	$E = \dfrac{1}{C}$

Mode	Parameter	Symbol	Equation
	mean airway pressure (cmH_2O) Note: PIP = peak inspiratory pressure, PEEP = positive end expiratory pressure, and k = 1.0 (for rectangular waveform) k = 0.5 (for triangular waveform) k = 0.5 to 1.0 (other waveforms)	$\overline{P}_{aw}$	$\overline{P}_{aw} = \left(\dfrac{1}{TCT}\right)\displaystyle\int_{t=0}^{t=TCT} P_{aw}\,dt$ $\overline{P}_{aw} = k(PIP - PEEP)\left(\dfrac{I}{I+E}\right)$ $\qquad + PEEP$ —
primary variables	pressure (cmH_2O)	P	Note: control of minute ventilation is important because it is a major determinant of gas exchange. Minute alveolar ventilation is usually adjusted to maintain an appropriate level of arterial carbon dioxide tension: $P_aCO_c \propto \dfrac{CO_2\ production}{\dot{V}_A}$
	volume (L)	V	
	flow ($cmH_2O/L/s$)	$\dot{V}$	
	time (seconds)	t	
	inspiratory time (seconds)	T_I	
	expiratory time (seconds)	T_E	
	frequency (breaths/min)	f	
	base of natural logarithm (≈ 2.72)	e	
	physiologic dead space volume (L)	V_D	

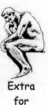

Extra for Experts

The equations for volume and flow were derived by solving the equation of motion using calculus. The equation of motion itself is not an algebraic equation, as it may appear, but rather a linear differential equation with constant coefficients (elastance and resistance). Its more technical form is

$$p(t) = E \cdot v(t) + R \cdot \frac{dv}{dt}$$

During volume control, if flow is constant (k) then the solution for $dv/dt = k$ is $v(t) = kt$. This says that volume as a function of time equals the constant flow times time. Thus, tidal volume is simply the constant (or average) flow times inspiratory time:

$$\left(V_T = \dot{V} \times T_I\right)$$

as shown in Table 4-1.

During pressure control, pressure, as a function of time is assumed constant. Thus $p(t)$ in the equation of motion becomes k and the equation is then solved to give the exponential equations for volume and flow shown in Table 4-1.

Mean airway pressure is defined as the average pressure at the airway opening over a given time interval, or as the area under the curve for one breathing cycle divided by the cycle time (inspiratory time plus expiratory time). It is generally higher for pressure controlled modes than volume controlled modes (at the same tidal volume) due to the differences in the shapes of the airway pressure waveforms (see Figure 4-4).

Figure 4-4. Comparison of volume control using a constant inspiratory flow (left) with pressure control using a constant inspiratory pressure (right). Shaded areas show pressure due to resistance. Unshaded areas show pressure due to compliance. The dashed line shows mean airway pressure. Note that lung volume and lung pressure have the same waveform shape.

Key Idea

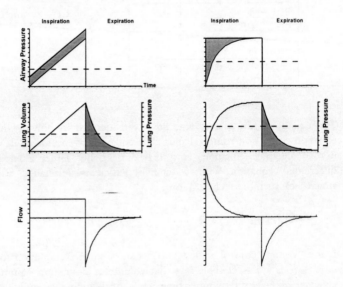

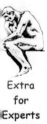

Infant ventilators have historically been designed as pressure controllers. This is because until recently, it has not been practical to measure and control very small tidal volumes and flows. In fact, most infant ventilators were little more than devices that generated a continuous flow that was intermittently switched between two pressure limiting valves; one for inspiratory pressure and one for PEEP. The fact that you can set the continuous flow on such ventilators has led to confusion among clinicians. Some think that the continuous flow setting on the ventilator is the inspiratory flow for mandatory breaths. For this reason, they tend to use lower flows for small neonates (say 6 L/min for infants weighing less than 1,000 grams) and higher flows (up to 12 or 15 L/min) for larger infants.

In reality, the continuous flow setting on an infant ventilator does nothing more than shape the inspiratory flow waveform (see Figures 3-3 and 3-4). The set flow is equal to the inspiratory flow only in the rare event that the pressure limit was set so high and the flow set so low that airway pressure never reaches the limit. This would result in essentially volume controlled ventilation as shown on the left in Figure 3-3.[1] More commonly, the flow is set high enough that the pressure limit is met early in inspiration if not instantly. The result is that the actual inspiratory flow will be a function of the pressure gradient (PIP − PEEP) and the patient's airway resistance (including endotracheal tube) and compliance. As you can see from Table 4-1, if the pressure waveform is rectangular:

$$\dot{V}_I = \left(\frac{\Delta P}{R} \right)\left(e^{-t/\tau}\right)$$

where $\dot{V}_I$ is inspiratory flow, ΔP is peak inspiratory pressure minus baseline pressure, R is respiratory system resistance, t is inspiratory time, τ is the respiratory system time constant (product of resistance and compliance) and e is a constant equal to about 2.72.

Peak inspiratory flow occurs when $t = 0$ (the start of inspiration) where the above equation simplifies to

---

[1] Hess D, Lind L. Nomograms for the application of the Bourns BP200 as a volume constant ventilator. Respir Care 1980; 26:248-250.

$$\dot{V}_I = \left(\frac{\Delta P}{R} \right)$$

from which we can see that peak inspiratory flow is determined only by the pressure settings and the resistance. If the pressure waveform is rounded rather than rectangular, the peak low is even less.

Key Idea

> The point of the above discussion is that the flow setting on an infant ventilator during pressure controlled modes is not the inspiratory flow entering the lungs and should be adjusted only as a way of shaping the pressure waveform.

It could even be argued that when flow is continuous rather than being delivered from a demand valve, it might be better to use higher rather than lower continuous flow settings, depending on the mechanical properties of the exhalation valve. If the valve has a linear resistance, than the higher the flow, the lower the resistance it will offer for a given PEEP level. Because the patient must divert flow from the exhalation valve for unassisted spontaneous inspirations, he is effectively breathing through the resistance of the exhalation valve. Thus, the higher the flow, the lower the valve resistance and the lower the imposed work of breathing.

The Time Constant

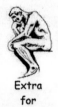

Extra
for
Experts

In Figure 4-4 you will note that the expiratory pressure and flow curves are the same shape for both volume and pressure control. This shape is called an exponential decay waveform (often mistakenly called a "decelerating" waveform), and it is characteristic of passive emptying of the lungs (exhalation). If the equation of motion is solved for lung pressure, we get the expression:

$$lung\ pressure\ during\ passive\ exhalation = \frac{tidal\ volume}{complinace} e^{-t/RC}$$

where e is the base of the natural logarithms (approximately 2.72), t is time (in this case the time allowed for exhalation), R is respiratory system resistance and C is respiratory system compliance. The product of R and C has units of time and is called the **time constant**, often symbolized by the Greek letter τ. It is referred to as a "constant" because for any value of R and C, the time constant always equals the time necessary for the lungs to empty by 63%. For example, when the expiratory time on a ventilator is set equal to the time constant, the patient will have passively exhaled only 63% of his tidal volume when the next breath starts. We can demonstrate this by setting t equal to RC:

$$lung\ pressure = \frac{tidal\ volume}{complinace}e^{-RC/RC} = \frac{tidal\ volume}{complinace}2.72^{-1} = \frac{tidal\ volume}{complinace}0.37$$

This expression shows that after an expiratory time equal to one time constant, only 37% of the lung pressure is left. Because volume is equal to pressure times compliance, we can multiply both sides of Equation 39-3 by compliance and see that only 37% of the tidal volume remains in the lungs. This implies that 63% of the tidal volume has been exhaled. After two time constants ($t = 2RC$), exhalation will be 87% completed and after 3 time constants, exhalation is 95% complete. After 5 time constants, exhalation is considered to be 100% complete for all practical purposes (Figure 4-5).

The time constant also governs volume and flow (as functions of time) during passive exhalation:

$$volume\ during\ exhalation = C \times \Delta P \times e^{-t/RC}$$

and

$$flow\ during\ exhalation = -\frac{\Delta P}{R}e^{-t/RC}$$

where R = resistance, C = compliance, and ΔP = the difference between end inspiratory pressure and end expiratory pressure (or [tidal volume ÷ compliance] - PEEP). Values for flow using this equation will be negative, signifying flow in the expiratory direction.

In more general terms, the time constant describes the passive behavior of a series connection of resistance and compliance in response to a step change in input pressure. A step change is a sudden change from one pressure to another. For exhalation, you can see in Figure 4-4 that pressure changes suddenly from peak inspiratory pressure to baseline pressure. This is true for both volume controlled and pressure controlled breaths. You might also notice that during pressure controlled ventilation with a rectangular pressure waveform, inspiration is also a step change in pressure. For this type of breath, the time constant can also be used to describe lung pressure, volume, and flow:

$$lung\ pressure\ during\ passive\ inhalation = \Delta P\left(1 - e^{-t/RC}\right)$$

$$volume = C \times \Delta P\left(1 - e^{-t/RC}\right)$$

$$flow = \frac{\Delta P}{R} e^{-t/RC}$$

Figure 4-5. Graph illustrating inspiratory and expiratory time constants.

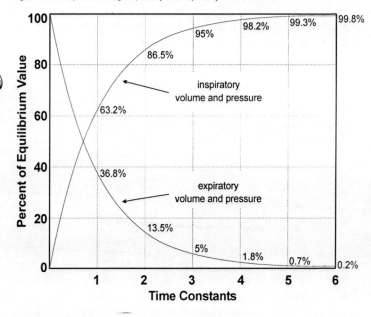

It is important to understand the concept of time constants in order to make appropriate ventilator setting adjustments. For example, in any mode of ventilation, the expiratory time should be at least 3 time constants long to avoid clinically important gas trapping. Similarly, in pressure controlled modes, inspiratory time should be at least 5 time constants long to get the maximum tidal volume from the set pressure gradient.

Understanding time constants, you can predict what will happen in various clinical situations. For example, in a pressure controlled mode, if resistance increases, the time constant increases, and it will take longer to deliver the same tidal volume. To compensate, you would have to increase either the inspiratory time or the inspiratory pressure limit. This is a qualitative prediction. You could also get quantitative predictions by programming a computer spreadsheet with the equations shown in Table 4-1. For example, you could enter the equation for tidal volume as a function of the pressure gradient, compliance inspiratory time and time constant. Then you could see the exact effect on tidal volume of changes in any of these variables. For instance, it is not immediately obvious how a large change in compliance might affect tidal volume. On the one hand, compliance determines the maximum tidal volume possible after 5 time constants have elapsed (maximum tidal volume = pressure gradient times compliance), so a larger compliance suggests that tidal volume should increase. On the other hand, the time constant itself is longer so the tidal volume will be less for any set inspiratory time. You would have to do the calculation to see which effect was greater.

Finally, a knowledge of time constants is required if you want to understand some of the new modes of ventilation that attempt to execute lung protective strategies. For example, the Hamilton Galileo measures the expiratory time constant of the patient and uses it to determine the IMV frequency that results in the least work of breathing. But it places a constraint on the frequency such that inspiratory time does not go below 1 time constant and expiratory time does not go below 2 time constants. This strategy is intended to minimize alveolar gas trapping (autoPEEP).

Review and Consider

1. If the tidal volume is 0.5 L and the frequency is 15 breaths/minute, what is the minute ventilation?

2. If the inspiratory time is 1.0 s and the I:E ratio is 1:2, what is the frequency?

3. On the Siemens Servo 900c ventilator, the operator can set minute ventilation and frequency. What happens to tidal volume if the frequency is increased?

4. Explain why mean inspiratory pressure (and hence mean airway pressure) is higher for volume control with a rectangular flow waveform than for pressure control with

a rectangular pressure waveform (assume tidal volumes and inspiratory times are the same).

5. Explain the meaning of the respiratory system time constant and why it is useful.

Questions 6-9 refer to pressure controlled ventilation with a rectangular pressure waveform

6. What happens to the driving pressure as you increase the pressure limit?

7. When ventilating a 1,500 gram neonate with respiratory distress syndrome, the pressure limit is 25 cmH_2O and PEEP is 5 cmH_2O. What is the maximum tidal volume (in mL/kg) achievable if compliance is 0.4 mL/ cmH_2O?

8. For the patient described above, what tidal volume is delivered if the inspiratory time is set at 0.6 seconds? Assume a time constant of 0.3 seconds.

9. What happens to mean airway pressure if you (A) increase the I:E ratio but do not change frequency, (B) increase the frequency but do not change the I:E ratio?

10. You are ventilating an adult patient with COPD in a VC-CMV mode. His compliance is 100 mL/cmH_2O and resistance 20 $cmH_2O/L/s$. The tidal volume is set at 500 mL, inspiratory flow is 60 L/min, and the ventilatory rate is 24 breaths/minute. Without looking at a graphics monitor, how could you determine if this patient might be exhibiting dynamic hyperinflation?

11. Why is arterial carbon dioxide tension (P_aCO_2) used to gauge the level of minute ventilation? *(Hint: see Table 4-1).*

Continuous Mandatory Ventilation (CMV)

Continuous mandatory ventilation (sometimes referred to as the "Assist/Control" mode) is intended to provide full ventilatory support. All breaths are mandatory. They are delivered by the ventilator at a preset volume or pressure, breath rate and inspiratory time. When people use the term "Assist/Control" they usually mean volume controlled CMV with "assist" referring to the possibility of patient triggering and "control" meaning that the patient becomes apneic, breaths will be machine triggered.

The ventilator will deliver a patient triggered breath if the patient has spontaneous inspiratory efforts, so it is important to set an appropriate trigger level. The ventilator delivers time triggered breaths if patient efforts are absent. The ventilator may **autotrigger** (repeatedly trigger itself when the trigger level is set too sensitive). As a result, hyperventilation, air trapping and patient anxiety often ensue. However, if the trigger level is not sensitive enough, the ventilator will not respond to the patient's inspiratory efforts, which results in an increased work of breathing. In the case where spontaneous triggering is counterproductive (if the patient tends to hyperventilate), sedation or paralysis may be required or another breathing pattern may be tried.

Volume Control

Indications

Theoretically, volume control (with a constant inspiratory flow) results in a more even distribution of ventilation (compared to pressure control) among lung units with different time constants where the units have equal resistances but unequal compliances (as in ARDS).[2] Volume controlled CMV is indicated when it is necessary to maintain precise regulation of minute ventilation or a blood gas parameter such as $PaCO_2$ in patients who have minimal respiratory drive such that synchrony with the ventilator is not a problem.

During VC-CMV, changes in the patient's lung mechanics result in changes in airway pressure. A reduction in lung compliance and or an increase in resistance will cause higher peak airway pressures. Care should also be taken to avoid setting a flow setting that fails to meet patient needs or exceeds their demand (if the patient is making inspiratory efforts). If the flow exceeds patient demands, inspiration may be prematurely shortened. An insufficient flow rate could result in an increase in the work of breathing and a concomitant increase in oxygen consumption. This would be visualized on a waveform monitor as the airway pressure dipping below baseline. To date, only one ventilator has software capable of avoiding this problem. The

---

[2] Respir Care 1994;(39)10:979-988.

Flow Augment feature of the Bear 1000 will increase the flow above the set value if the patient's inspiratory effort causes airway pressure to go below baseline.

Example

Perhaps the most common application of this mode of ventilation is to facilitate therapeutic hyperventilation in the patient with traumatic brain injury. Patients are often sedated to reduce oxygen consumption, ventilator asynchrony, and to minimize the patient's response to noxious stimuli. VC-CMV can achieve precise regulation of $PaCO_2$ and support efforts to alleviate intracranial hypertension and reduce the likelihood of secondary complications from cerebral ischemia.

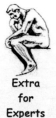

**Extra
for
Experts**

Exactly how you would manage the ventilator to regulate $PaCO_2$? Let's assume you have a 40 kg pediatric victim of an automobile accident with head trauma. Initial settings on VC-CMV are frequency = 15/min, tidal volume = 200 mL which yield a $PaCO_2$ of 37 torr (mm Hg). The physician requests that the $PaCO_2$ be held between 30 and 35 torr. What do you do?

The first thing you must know is the relation between $PaCO_2$ and minute ventilation. In Table 4-1 we see that $PaCO_2$ is directly proportional to metabolic carbon dioxide production and inversely proportional to alveolar ventilation. The exact equation is:

$$P_aCO_2 = \frac{\dot{V}CO_2 \times (P_B - P_AH_2O)}{\dot{V}_A}$$

where P_aCO_2 is the partial pressure of carbon dioxide in arterial blood, $\dot{V}CO_2$ is carbon dioxide production, P_B is the barometric pressure, P_AH_2O is the partial pressure of water vapor in the alveoli, and $\dot{V}_A$ is alveolar ventilation.

Because our patient's current P_aCO_2 is too high, we know from the equation that we must increase the $\dot{V}_A$, but how much? If we multiply both sides of the equation by $\dot{V}_A$ we get:

$$\dot{V}_A \times P_aCO_2 = \dot{V}CO_2 \times (P_B - P_AH_2O)$$

Over short periods, we can assume that carbon dioxide production remains constant. If the weather is stable we can assume that $(P_B - P_A H_2 O)$ also stays constant. If the whole right hand side of the equation stays constant, then we conclude that as $\dot{V}_A$ increases, $P_a CO_2$ must decrease and vice versa. We can relate two sets of $\dot{V}_A$ and $P_a CO_2$ (corresponding to old and new ventilator settings) as follows:

$$old\,\dot{V}_A \times old\,P_a CO_2 = \dot{V}CO_2 \times (P_B - P_A H_2 O)$$

$$new\,\dot{V}_A \times new\,P_a CO_2 = \dot{V}CO_2 \times (P_B - P_A H_2 O)$$

Because we are assuming that the right hand side of the equation stays constant between old and new settings we can say that:

$$old\,\dot{V}_A \times old\,P_a CO_2 = new\,\dot{V}_A \times new\,P_a CO_2$$

From Table 4-1 we see that alveolar ventilation is the product of ventilatory frequency and alveolar volume (which is tidal volume minus dead space volume). If dead space volume remains constant, we can rewrite the above equation as:

$$old\,f \times (old\,V_T - V_D) \times old\,P_a CO_2 = new\,f \times (new\,V_T - V_D) \times new\,P_a CO_2$$

where V_T is tidal volume and V_D is dead space volume. Dead space volume us usually estimated as 1.0 mL/kg body weight. We now have everything we need to precisely adjust our patient's $PaCO_2$ by changing the frequency, the tidal volume, or both.

The patient's tidal volume is only 200 mL/40 kg = 5 mL/kg. If there is no significant lung damage but the PaO_2 seems a little low, we might choose to increase tidal volume instead of frequency. Because the old and new frequency will be the same, the above equation can be rearranged and simplified to:

$$new\,V_T = \frac{(old\,V_T - V_D) \times old\,P_a CO_2}{new\,P_a CO_2} + V_D$$

We want the new PaO_2 to be between 30 and 35 mm Hg, so we pick 33 mm Hg to put into the equation along with an estimated dead space of 40 kg x 1 mL/kg = 40 mL:

$$new\,V_T = \frac{(200-40)\times 37}{33} + 40 \approx 219\,mL$$

Therefore, to reduce the patient's PaO_2 from 37 torr to 33 torr, we must increase the tidal volume from 200 mL to 219 mL.

Suppose the patient also has a lung contusion and we wish to minimize further damage from the ventilator. Instead of increasing the tidal volume, we would increase the frequency. In this case, the equation is even simpler:

$$new\,f = \frac{old\,f \times old\,P_aCO_2}{new\,P_aCO_2}$$

Using the patient's current frequency and PaO_2 along with the same desired PaO_2 we get:

$$new\,f = \frac{15\times 37}{33} = 16.8 \approx 17\,breaths\,/\,min$$

Thus, if we increase the ventilatory rate from 15 to 17 breaths per minute we should get a PaO_2 very close to 33 torr.

Pressure Control

Indications

Theoretically, pressure control (with a constant inspiratory pressure) results in a more even distribution of ventilation (compared to volume control) among lung units with different time constants when units have equal compliances but unequal resistances (as in status asthmaticus).[2] Pressure controlled CMV is indicated when adequate oxygenation has been difficult to achieve in volume controlled modes of ventilation or for patients who have difficulty synchronizing with the ventilator. Also, the instability of tidal volume caused by intermittent airway leaks can be minimized by using pressure controlled ventilation rather than volume controlled ventilation.[3] Increased tidal volume stability may lead to better gas exchange and lower risk of pulmonary volutrauma (damage caused by stretching the tissue beyond its elastic limit by using too large a delivered volume).

---

[3] Respir Care 1996;41(8):728-735.

Use of a rectangular pressure waveform opens alveoli earlier in the inspiratory phase during PC-CMV and results in a higher mean airway pressure than VC-CMV with a rectangular flow waveform. This allows more time for oxygenation to occur. As with VC-CMV, gas exchange is more predictable than modes that provide partial ventilatory support (like intermittent mandatory ventilation). In PC-CMV however, inspiratory flow is not preset by the clinician. It is variable and dependent on patient effort and lung mechanics, thus improving patient comfort and patient-ventilator synchrony.

Because tidal volume is not directly controlled, the pressure gradient (PIP – PEEP) is the primary parameter used to alter the breath size and hence carbon dioxide tensions. Typically, the peak inspiratory pressure (PIP) is adjusted to provide the patient with a tidal volume within the desired range while PEEP is changed less frequently. As with VC-CMV, the mandatory breath rate set by the clinician is dependent upon the presence of ventilatory muscle activity and the severity of lung disease. When higher mandatory breath rates are needed (30 – 60 breaths per minute), it is essential for the clinician to provide a sufficient expiratory time to prevent dynamic hyperinflation.

As long as lung mechanics and patient effort remain constant, the volume and peak flow delivered to the patient will remain unchanged. Should a decrease in patient effort occur (or a decrease in compliance or an increase in resistance), less volume will be delivered for the pre-set pressure gradient. Conversely, improvements in patient effort and mechanics can dramatically increase the volume delivery to the patient in this mode. Close tidal volume monitoring is required to avoid ventilator-induced hypoventilation or lung damage due to over expansion with too large of an end inspiratory volume (**volutrauma**).

Key Idea

> Volutrauma can be caused by too large a tidal volume or a normal tidal volume on top of too large an end-expiratory volume due to too much PEEP.

Example

Perhaps the most common use of PC-CMV has been in patients with ARDS whose oxygenation status has failed to improve with the application of VC-CMV. It is sometimes argued that pressure controlled ventilation is superior to volume controlled ventilation because it results in lower peak pressure. Peak transrespiratory pressure during volume control is higher because of the resistive pressure drop across the endotracheal tube and upper airways (pressure drop equals flow times resistance, in the equation of motion). However, it is a high transalveolar pressure (lung or alveolar pressure – pleural pressure) that leads to lung damage, not necessarily a high transrespiratory system pressure (pressure at airway opening – pressure on body surface). For example, a high peak transrespiratory pressure could result if the patient has severely decreased chest wall compliance or a partially blocked endotracheal tube, but the transalveolar pressure would be normal. If tidal volumes are the same for pressure control and volume control, then both would produce the same peak alveolar pressure, and presumably the same risk for over-distention.

PC-CMV with an inverse I:E ratio (I is greater than E) is called Pressure Controlled Inverse Ratio Ventilation or Airway Pressure Release Ventilation. The idea is to maintain lung inflation as long as possible using long inspiratory times and short expiratory times, but allow the patient to superimpose spontaneous breaths on the long mandatory breaths. Usually these breaths are allowed to promote patient comfort but they are not very effective for ventilation. Thus, the pressure gradient must be high enough to allow the patient an effective mandatory tidal volume. The patient's oxygen delivery should be closely monitored because this form of ventilation results in a high mean airway pressure that may impair cardiac output.

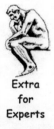

Extra
for
Experts

Suppose you have a patient who is not doing well on VC-CMV. You decide to switch him to PC-CMV with hopes of improving oxygenation. You need to select the pressure limit and inspiratory time carefully or you will have ventilation problems (high arterial carbon dioxide tension) on top of oxygenation problems. What values should you select for the pressure limit and inspiratory time so that you deliver the same tidal volume?

To answer this question you must know the patient's compliance and inspiratory time constant, which means you must also know his resistance. The idea is to calculate the desired pressure limit and inspiratory time rather than attempt to find them by trial and error on an unstable patient. If you are lucky, the ventilator will display compliance, resistance and the time constant for you. If you have an older ventilator, you must calculate them by hand. Fortunately, using an inspiratory hold during volume control you can collect all the data you need.

Let's say the patient's tidal volume is 600 mL and inspiratory flow is 60 L/min (1 L/s) with resulting peak pressure of 50 cm H_2O, static or plateau pressure of 40 cm H_2O, mean pressure of 28 cm H_2O, and PEEP of 10 cm H_2O. We know that compliance is the ratio of volume change (ie, tidal volume) to static pressure change associated with elastic recoil only, excluding the pressure component due to flow resistance. The inspiratory hold gives us that static pressure change because flow goes to zero, as shown in Figure 3-7 (ie, static pressure change = plateau pressure minus PEEP). Thus, we estimate compliance as:

$$compliance = \frac{tidal\ volume}{P_{plateau} - PEEP} = \frac{600}{40 - 10} = 20\ mL\ /\ cmH_2O$$

We also know that resistance is the ratio of flow change (ie, set inspiratory flow) to the dynamic pressure change associated with gas moving through the airways. This pressure change is not available directly from the ventilator display. However, from the equation of motion we recall that inspiratory pressure at each moment is the sum of elastic and resistive components. We know the elastic component at one particular moment, end inspiration ($P_{plateau}$ − PEEP). We also know total airway pressure at that same moment (peak inspiratory pressure, PIP). Therefore, the dynamic pressure change we need must be the difference between the two and resistance is thus:

$$resistance = \frac{PIP - P_{plateau}}{inspiratory\ flow} = \frac{50 - 40}{1} = 10\ cmH_2O \cdot s \cdot L^{-1}$$

Now we can calculate the time constant, τ, making sure to convert the compliance from mL/ cm H_2O to L/ cm H_2O so that the units are consistent with those of resistance.

$$\tau = RC = \frac{0.02L}{cmH_2O} \times \frac{10\ cmH_2O \cdot s}{L} = 0.2\ s$$

Back to the original question: What pressure limit do we use to get a tidal volume of 600 mL? If compliance is the ratio of volume change to pressure change, then the pressure change must be the ratio of the tidal volume and the estimated compliance. Recognizing that static pressure is the plateau pressure during volume control but it is the peak inspiratory pressure (ie, pressure limit) during pressure control, we have:

$$PIP - PEEP = \frac{tidal\ volume}{compliance} = \frac{600\ mL}{20\ mL\,/\,cmH_2O} = 30\ cmH_2O$$

Because PEEP = 10 cm H_2O,

$$PIP = 30\ cmH_2O + PEEP = 30 + 10 = 40\ cmH_2O$$

Recall from our discussion of limit variables in Chapter 3 that the peak pressure for mandatory breaths is measured relative to atmospheric pressure. Therefore, you would set the pressure limit to 40 cm H_2O to get a tidal volume of 600 mL.

Now that I have dragged you through this whole ordeal, I'll tell you a secret: just set the pressure limit during pressure control equal to the plateau pressure during volume control. Of course, now you know why.

But we are not finished yet. The ventilator will only deliver 600 mL if the 40 cm H_2O is maintained long enough. From our prior discussion about time constants, we recall that the maximum tidal volume during pressure control will be delivered when inspiratory time is about 5 time constants long. With an estimated time constant of 0.2 seconds, our patient will require an inspiratory time of 1.0 second.

Note that if you had been using Pressure Support (which is measured relative to PEEP) to deliver the same volume for spontaneous breaths, the pressure limit (and hence the peak inspiratory pressure) would be 50 cm H_2O (ie, set Pressure Support level of 40 cm H_2O to deliver the 600 mL plus the PEEP of 10 cm H_2O).

Dual Control

Indications

Dual controlled CMV is indicated in patients with moderate to severe lung disease, in which unstable pulmonary mechanics make precise control of minute ventilation difficult to achieve. In DC-CMV, the ventilator attempts to maintain a preset tidal volume and/or pressure limit in response to changing patient conditions.

On the Dräger Evita 4 ventilator, Continuous Mandatory Ventilation + Autoflow is an example of a DC-CMV mode. The tidal volume, breath rate and maximum (alarm) pressure limit are operator preset. Once connected to the ventilator, the patient-ventilator interaction that occurs in the first few breaths is critical. Initially, the ventilator calculates total system compliance. On the succeeding breaths, the ventilator monitors the peak airway pressures and expiratory tidal volume. The ventilator then determines the pressure limit necessary to deliver the clinician set "target" tidal volume, for the given total system compliance. (again, we say "target" because the ventilator aims to deliver it, over the course of several breaths, but may not hit the mark if the alarm pressure threshold is exceeded). If the patient's lung compliance improves (or patient effort increases), the ventilator delivers subsequent mandatory breaths at a lower pressure limit to maintain the target tidal volume. This reduces the risk of alveolar over-distention. However, it may also reduce support when the patient still needs it if the ventilator interprets anxiety-driven hyperventilation as an improved patient condition.

Conversely, the ventilator responds to worsening pulmonary compliance (or decreasing patient effort) by increasing the pressure limit until the tidal volume is achieved. The ventilator makes pressure limit changes in small increments, $3 - 4$ cmH$_2$O per breath, and will not exceed the maximum pressure limit set by the operator.

Example

DC-CMV has been used in infants with RDS after administration of surfactant. Rapidly changing pulmonary mechanics from surfactant administration are associated with complications such as pulmonary air leaks, intraventricular hemorrhage and bronchopulmonary dysplasia. DC-CMV adapts to changes in a patient's lung mechanics and may result in a lower incidence of these common complications.

Review and Consider

12. If there were a significant leak through a bronchopleural fistula, which mode would minimize the effect of the lost tidal volume, VC-CMV or PC-CMV?

13. For a patient with atelectasis and problems with oxygenation, would you prefer VC-CMV or PC-CMV?

14. What does the term "Assist/Control" usually mean?

15. For a given tidal volume and compliance, which mode of ventilation results in the lowest peak alveolar pressure, VC-CMV or PC-CMV?

16. The terms "volutrauma" (injury due to volume) and "barotrauma" (injury due to pressure) refer to the damage done to the lungs when they are overstretched. Why is volutrauma a more accurate word?

17. Why might DC-CMV be more likely to meet an infant's ventilatory needs after surfactant administration than conventional PC-CMV?

18. What happens to the level of ventilatory support when the patient increases his inspiratory efforts due to dyspnea during DC-CMV? What might be the clinical consequences?

Intermittent Mandatory Ventilation (IMV)

IMV is a partial support mode that requires the patient to sustain some of the work of breathing. The level of mechanical support needed is dependent upon the presence and degree of ventilatory muscle weakness, and severity of lung disease. In this mode, mandatory breaths are delivered at a set rate. Between the mandatory breaths, the patient can breathe spontaneously.

When the mandatory breath is patient triggered, it is commonly referred to as synchronized IMV (SIMV). With synchronized intermittent mandatory ventilation (SIMV), the ventilator will coordinate the start of inspiratory flow with the patient's inspiratory effort. If no spontaneous efforts occur, the ventilator will deliver a time triggered breath.

Because spontaneous breaths decrease pleural pressure, ventilatory support with IMV usually results in a lower mean intrathoracic pressure than CMV, which can result in a higher cardiac output.

When used to wean a patient from mechanical ventilation, the intent of IMV is to provide respiratory muscle rest during the mandatory breaths and exercise during spontaneous breaths. However, studies have demonstrated that IMV weaning prolongs the duration of mechanical ventilation when compared to Pressure Support ventilation and spontaneous breathing trials.[4]

The basic idea behind IMV is that the ventilator watches the patient and if he does not generate a spontaneous breath within a certain time widow, the ventilator will step in and generate a mandatory breath. You can think of the ventilator as sort of a watchdog to make sure the patient maintains an adequate minute ventilation. Carrying this idea a little further, we get a unique form of IMV called **Mandatory Minute Ventilation**. In this mode, the ventilator takes a more general view of the patient and monitors the exhaled minute ventilation. As long as the patient either triggers mandatory breaths or generates his own spontaneous breath often enough to maintain a preset minute ventilation, the ventilator does not interfere. However, if the exhaled minute ventilation falls below the operator set value, the ventilator will trigger mandatory breaths (in volume control) or increase the pressure limit (in pressure control) until the target is reached.

Volume Control

Indications

Volume controlled IMV is indicated for patients with relatively normal lung function recovering from sedation or rapidly reversing respiratory failure.

As the patient is capable of providing more work, the level of ventilatory support can be decreased accordingly. Weaning from VC-IMV usually involves the gradual reduction of the mandatory breath rate, while maintaining a constant tidal volume. Frequency is decreased rather than tidal volume because patients' spontaneous breaths tend to be shallow at first and relatively large mandatory breaths tend to prevent atelectasis and preserve oxygenation. Another reason is that as the patient's spontaneous efforts begin to support a normal tidal volume it could cause an increased work of breathing if the ventilator delivered breaths that were too small. When the mandatory breath rate has been reduced enough (around 4 breaths per minute) the patient is assessed for either a spontaneous breathing trial or extubation.

---

[4] Evidence-based guidelines for weaning and discontinuing ventilatory support. Respir Care 2002;47(1):69-90.

Example

VC-IMV is usually selected for patients with neuromuscular disorders, such as Guillian-Barre syndrome. These patients typically have normal lung function and an intact ventilatory drive. As the disease progresses, muscle weakness eventually affects the patient's ventilatory muscles. Mechanical ventilation is considered when it difficult for the patient to sustain tidal volumes and minute ventilation. Large tidal volumes (12 to 15 mL/kg) and high peak flows (> 60 L/M) may be needed to alleviate dyspnea and maximize patient comfort. As respiratory muscle function improves, mandatory breath support can be reduced.

Pressure Control

Indications

Pressure controlled IMV is indicated when preservation of the patient's spontaneous efforts is important but adequate oxygenation has been difficult to achieve with volume controlled modes. PC-IMV has been traditionally associated with mechanical ventilation of infants, not only because of their oxygenation problems but also because it is difficult to control tidal volumes at such small values.

Liberation from this mode involves the gradual reduction of the peak inspiratory pressure, as well as the mandatory breath rate. As lung compliance improves, adjustments in peak inspiratory pressure and set mandatory breath rate are critical to prevent volutrauma and hyperventilation.

Example

Perhaps the most familiar scenario is the application of pressure controlled IMV in premature infants with RDS (respiratory distress syndrome). Initially, because of a noncompliant lung, compliant chest wall and poor respiratory effort, the infant may require a relatively high peak inspiratory pressure and mandatory breath rate to achieve acceptable tidal volumes and acid base balance. Liberation from this mode of partial support ventilation involves the gradual reduction of the peak inspiratory pressure, as well as the mandatory breath rate. It is important to monitor tidal volumes because the improving compliance may lead to lung over-distention at pressure limits that had previously been acceptable.

Dual Control

Indications

As a partial support mode of ventilation, dual controlled IMV is useful in stabilizing tidal volume on spontaneous and mandatory breaths in patients with changing pulmonary mechanics or inconsistent respiratory efforts. The key point with this mode of ventilation, as with any partial ventilatory support mode, is to allow spontaneous breaths to occur.

In DC-IMV, the clinician sets the mandatory breath rate, maximum inspiratory pressure limit and tidal volume (and for within-breath dual control modes, inspiratory flow). Caution should be exercised with setting the peak flow for within-breath dual control, such as when using P_{max} on the Dräger Evita 4. As with a volume control mode, the clinician should adjust the flow to match the patient's inspiratory demands. Care should be taken to ensure appropriate inspiratory times and I:E ratios are achieved. Failure to do so, on mandatory breaths, will result in flows that either fail to meet or exceed a patient's demands. An increased work of breathing and concomitant increase in oxygen consumption may result. Furthermore, inappropriate flow settings will defeat the benefits of dual control; if flow is too high the breath is essentially volume controlled and if too low inspiratory time may be prolonged.

Example

A clinical application of this mode of ventilation would be in a patient with pneumonia and rapidly changing lung mechanics due to intermittent secretion problems. In VC-IMV the constant tidal volume may cause regional over-distention and further injure the lungs. Changing ventilatory drive may make the set inspiratory flow inappropriate much of the time, leading to asynchrony and increased work of breathing. PC-IMV would be even worse because the changing lung compliance and resistance would frequently lead to under- or over-ventilation and unstable blood gases. DC-IMV maintains a consistent tidal volume as lung mechanics change, stabilizing gas exchange while protecting the lungs.

Review and Consider

19. What is the difference between IMV and SIMV? Why would SIMV be more important in PC-IMV than VC-IMV?

20. What is the difference between CMV and IMV in terms of adverse cardiac effects?

21. IMV is still widely used as a weaning mode. Does the currently available evidence suggest that this is the best practice?

22. What is the difference between IMV and Mandatory Minute Ventilation?

23. When would you use VC-IMV instead of PC-IMV?

24. Why has $\overline{\text{PC}}$-IMV been used historically for neonates instead of VC-IMV?

25. If Mandatory Minute Ventilation automatically adjusts the support given by the ventilator in response to the patient's needs, why would we need DC-IMV?

Continuous Spontaneous Ventilation (CSV)

Pressure Control

Spontaneous breath modes include those in which all breaths are initiated and ended by the patient. The level of support determines the patient's work of breathing. Continuous positive airway pressure (CPAP), Pressure Support, Proportional Assist and Automatic Tube Compensation are examples of continuous spontaneous breath modes, specifically, PC-CSV.

CPAP provides no direct assistance in the work of breathing. Rather, it helps to maintain an adequate functional residual lung volume that may improve lung compliance. Improving lung compliance may reduce the muscular effort the patient needs to breathe. If CPAP levels are set too high, reduced lung compliance may result, or the diaphragm may be lowered such that the mechanical advantage is reduced. This could lead to an increased work of breathing. In addition, high CPAP could lead to a reduced cardiac output. Depending on the ventilator, CPAP may be delivered as simply a constant flow source from which the patient breathes without any ventilator interaction or it may be delivered with a demand valve. Demand valve breaths are patient triggered, pressure limited (at the CPAP pressure or very slightly above it) and either pressure or flow cycled.

Pressure Support is a form of PC-CSV that does assist inspiratory efforts. Breaths are patient triggered, pressure limited, and flow cycled. Because the patient has control over the frequency, duration, and size of the breath, synchrony and comfort are improved. At very low levels of support, this mode compensates for the resistive work of breathing through an endotracheal tube. At higher levels, the ventilator may assume all of the work of breathing. High levels of support reduce the respiratory rate, decrease respiratory muscle fatigue, lower oxygen consumption, and improve or stabilize spontaneous tidal volumes. However, the positive attributes of this mode of ventilation can be negated if ventilator parameters are not properly set. It is critical that the trigger sensitivity be set correctly. Of equal importance is the clinician-set rise time (the time required for the ventilator to reach the inspiratory pressure limit). Ventilator graphics are often helpful when adjusting this parameter and optimizing patient-ventilator synchrony. A rise time that is too short may result in pressure overshoot and prematurely cycle the breath off. A rise time that is too long may not give the patient enough peak flow and prolong inspiration.

Proportional Assist is a unique mode that may provide the ultimate in patient synchrony. Each breath is patient triggered, pressure limited and flow cycled similar to Pressure Support. However, the pressure limit is not set at some constant, arbitrary value. Rather, it is automatically adjusted by the ventilator to be proportional to the patient's effort. The idea of this mode of ventilation is to allow the ventilator to support, and essentially cancel, the specific effects of pulmonary pathology. That is, the ventilator can be set to support either the extra elastance or the extra resistance (or both) caused by lung disease.

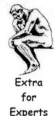

To understand this, we start with the form of the equation of motion describing spontaneous breathing:

$$P_{mus} = E_{normal} \times volume + R_{noirmal} \times flow$$

When pathology increases elastance and/or resistance, the equation becomes:

$$P_{mus} = \left(E_{normal} + E_{abnormal}\right) \times volume + \left(R_{normal} + R_{abnormal}\right) \times flow$$

The above equation can be rearranged to show the normal and abnormal loads. Recall that load, in this context, is the pressure to overcome either elastance or resistance (elastance times volume = pressure; resistance times flow = pressure).

$$P_{mus} = \left(E_{normal} \times volume\right) + \left(E_{abnormal} \times volume\right)$$
$$+ \left(R_{normal} \times flow\right) + \left(R_{abnormal} \times flow\right)$$

or equivalently,

$$P_{mus} = \left(E_{normal} \times volume\right) + \left(abnormal\ elastic\ load\right)$$
$$+ \left(R_{normal} \times flow\right) + \left(abnormal\ resistive\ load\right)$$

The abnormal elastic load and the abnormal resistive load (which have units of pressure) can be added together to get the total abnormal load.

$$P_{mus} = \left(E_{normal} \times volume\right) + \left(R_{normal} \times flow\right) + \left(abnormal\ load\right)$$

So finally, we see that the patient must support both the normal and abnormal loads:

$$P_{mus} = \left(normal\ load\right) + \left(abnormal\ load\right)$$

The last equation implies that in the presence of increased load due to abnormal elastance and/or resistance, the muscle pressure must increase to provide the same (normal) tidal volume and flow. If we want to mechanically support the abnormal load, and allow muscle pressure to fall back to normal levels (sometimes called "unloading the muscles"), all we have to do is let the ventilator generate pressure equal to the abnormal load. So the equation becomes

$$P_{mus} + P_{vent} = \left(normal\ load\right) + \left(abnormal\ load\right)$$

How much pressure must the ventilator generate to support the abnormal load?

Isolating P_{vent} in the above equation we get:

$$P_{vent} = abnormal\ load = E_{abnormal} \times volume + R_{abnormal} \times flow$$

During Proportional Assist, the ventilator monitors volume and flow and generates airway pressure proportional to each, using $E_{abnormal}$ and $R_{abnormal}$ as constants of proportionality. In engineering terms, these constants are gain (or amplification) factors set on the volume and flow signals. In practice, the ventilator measures airway pressure and flow. The flow signal is integrated to get a volume signal. The flow and volume signals are fed through two amplifiers and through a mixer (that combines the amplified signals). The mixed signal is fed to a pressure generator (such as a piston) connected to the patient's airway. The ventilator's control circuit is programmed with the equation of motion, so that each moment, airway pressure is controlled to be equal to the amplified volume signal plus the amplified flow signal. The gain of the flow amplifier is set to the abnormal resistance and the gain of the volume amplifier is set to the abnormal elastance, assuming these values have been estimated beforehand by the operator. Thus, the specific mechanical abnormality of the patient is supported. In effect, the abnormal load is eliminated and the patient *perceives* only normal ventilatory load. This is analogous to power steering on an automobile, making driving easier while maintaining complete responsiveness to the operator's motions. No ventilator power is wasted forcing the patient to breathe in an unnatural pattern, as can happen with pressure support. This makes proportional assist potentially the most comfortable mode of ventilation yet designed.

At the time of this writing, Proportional Assist is only available on ventilators sold outside the United States due to the delays associated with getting new modes cleared by the Food and Drug Administration. What has been approved is a sort of partial implementation called **Automatic Tube Compensation**. This feature allows the operator to enter the size of the patient's endotracheal tube and have the ventilator calculate the tube's resistance and generate pressure to compensate for the abnormal resistive load:

$$P_{vent} = abnormal\ resistive\ load = R_{tube} \times flow^2$$

Note that in this equation, the ventilator pressure is proportional to *flow squared* because that is a better model of the turbulent flow in the upper airways.

Indications

PC-CSV ventilation is indicated to reduce the work of breathing and improve or stabilize oxygenation by reducing alveolar collapse in patients that do not require full ventilatory support.

Example

An example of the use of pressure controlled CSV is nasal CPAP in the preterm surfactant deficient infant with respiratory distress syndrome to prevent the need for intubation. CPAP holds open collapsible small airways, and surfactant deficient alveoli. As a result, alveolar gas exchange is enhanced.

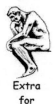

Extra for Experts

Another common example of PC-CSV is the Pressure Support mode found on most ventilators. Often, this mode is set at a low level (5 to 10 cmH$_2$O) to approximately compensate for the resistive load imposed by the endotracheal tube. Of course, Automatic Tube Compensation is a more accurate way to do this while providing PC-CSV.

Suppose you don't have the option of Automatic Tube Compensation and you want to set Pressure Support as accurately as possible to compensate for the resistive load of the endotracheal tube. How would you select the pressure limit? Recall that load has units of pressure, so in theory we set the Pressure Support level equal to the resistive load. Recall further that resistive load is calculated as flow times resistance. Assuming that we can get the patient's respiratory system resistance (which is mostly the resistance of the endotracheal tube) either from the ventilator's display or by hand calculation (see Extra for Experts in the Pressure Control section above). We are still left with the problem of choosing a value for inspiratory flow. One approach would be to estimate average inspiratory flow by measuring the patient's spontaneous tidal volume and dividing by his inspiratory time. Assuming a sick patient probably has an I:E ratio of about 1:1, you can estimate inspiratory time (T_I in seconds) from the observed spontaneous breathing frequency, (f, in breaths/minute) as:

$$T_I \approx \frac{60}{2 \times f}$$

If you can't measure a spontaneous tidal volume, you can estimate it from the Radford Nomogram (Figure 4-2) using the patient's weight and spontaneous breath rate.

An easier way is to use the patient's peak inspiratory flow for spontaneous breaths, if the ventilator can measure and display it. Using peak rather than mean inspiratory flow may slightly overestimate the required Pressure Support, but it probably makes no clinical difference.

Dual Control

Indications

Dual controlled CSV is indicated to stabilize minute ventilation in spontaneously breathing patients with an intact but perhaps variable ventilatory drive and normal pulmonary mechanics. As a spontaneous breathing mode, all breaths are patient triggered, pressure limited and flow-cycled. The patient controls the inspiratory time, tidal volume, inspiratory flow and frequency. The clinician sets a target tidal volume. The ventilator monitors exhaled volume and frequency and regulates, on a breath-by-breath basis, the actual pressure limit needed to meet the set volume. The Volume Support ventilation mode on the Siemens Servo 300 is an example of DC-CSV.

Example

The application of DC-CSV may be best suited to post-operative patients with normal respiratory systems. These patients require intubation for airway protection and short-term mechanical ventilation to support inconsistent spontaneous minute ventilation. As they recover from anesthesia, the ventilator senses their increased inspiratory force and reduces the pressure limit such that weaning is automatic.

Review and Consider

26. Why are all CSV modes pressure controlled rather than volume controlled?

27. If CPAP and Pressure Support are patient triggered, pressure limited, and patient cycled, why are they considered different modes?

28. What is the difference between Proportional Assist and Automatic Tube Compensation?

29. Setting parameters for Proportional Assist is completely different than for any other mode. For other modes, we could look up appropriate tidal volumes and frequencies from tables like the Radford Nomogram. This is not true for Proportional Assist. Explain.

30. Explain why Proportional Assist may provide the ultimate in patient synchrony.

31. What is the difference between setting Pressure Support at a low level and using Automatic Tube Compensation? Why use either?

Self Assessment Questions

Definitions

- Pressure rise time

- Mean airway pressure

- Time constant

- Autotrigger

- Volutrauma

- Mandatory minute ventilation

- Proportional Assist

- Automatic Tube Compensation

True or False

1. The primary variable we wish to control when a patient is connected to a ventilator is minute ventilation.

2. Figure 4-1 shows that if you know inspiratory time and inspiratory flow, you can calculate tidal volume.

3. Table 4-1 shows that minute exhaled ventilation is larger than minute alveolar ventilation.

4. Minute ventilation is more stable with pressure control modes than volume control modes.

5. Mean inspiratory pressure is generally higher for volume control than pressure control at the same tidal volume and inspiratory time.

6. The time constant varies depending on whether you are considering pressure, volume, or flow waveforms.

7. Knowledge of the time constant helps in making appropriate ventilator settings.

8. The term "Assist/Control" is often used to mean volume controlled SIMV.

9. Volume control results in a more even distribution of ventilation than pressure control when lung units have equal resistances but unequal compliances.

10. Pressure control results in a more even distribution of ventilation than pressure control when lung units have equal compliances but unequal resistances.

11. During PC-CMV, increasing PEEP will decrease the tidal volume.

12. PC-CMV results in a lower peak inspiratory pressure than VC-CMV and thus reduces the risk of volutrauma.

13. PC-CMV results in a higher mean airway pressure than VC-CMV which may impair cardiac output.

14. DC-CMV will reduce the level of ventilatory support if the patient increases her breathing rate due to anxiety.

15. CMV implies full ventilatory support while IMV implies partial ventilatory support.

16. IMV results in a higher mean intrathoracic pressure than CMV.

17. VC-IMV is more often used for patients with normal lungs whereas PC-IMV is more frequently used for patients with lung disease.

18. In some forms of DC-IMV, the clinician must set flow as well as volume, and pressure criteria.

19. Improper balancing of pressure, volume, and flow settings can defeat the purpose of dual control within breaths.

20. CPAP is a form of assisted ventilation classified as PC-CSV.

21. Proportional assist theoretically allows the ventilator to support the abnormal load due to lung pathology and to preserve the patient's ability to support his own normal load.

22. Automatic Tube Compensation provides pressure in proportion to the patient's inspiratory flow demand.

23. If a patient stops triggering breaths in the DC-CSV mode, he will hypoventilate.

Multiple Choice

1. Minute ventilation is directly controlled by:

    a. Inspiratory time and tidal volume

    b. Tidal volume and inspiratory flow

    c. Tidal volume and ventilatory frequency

    d. Cycle time and I:E ratio

2. According to Figure 4-2, the appropriate tidal volume for a 10 kg child breathing at a frequency of 30 breaths/minute is:

    a. 30 mL

    b. 25 mL

    c. 35 mL

    d. not enough information to tell

3. According to Figure 4-3, all of the following factors affect mean airway pressure during pressure controlled ventilation except:

    a. The shape of the pressure waveform.

    b. The pressure gradient.

    c. The I:E ratio.

    d. The time constant of the respiratory system.

4. According to Figure 4-3, which of the following are not true: ___

    a. Lung pressure and lung volume have the same waveshape.

    b. Volume control results in a higher mean airway pressure than pressure control.

    c. Peak inspiratory flow is higher for pressure control.

    d. Peak expiratory flow is the same for volume control and pressure control.

5. According to Table 4-1, tidal volume during pressure control is determined by all of the following except:

    a. Pressure gradient

    b. I:E ratio

    c. Compliance

    d. Time constant

    e. Inspiratory time

6. Knowledge of time constants is useful for all of the following except:

    a. Predicting inspiratory volume during pressure controlled ventilation.

    b. Predicting gas trapping.

    c. Understanding lung protective strategies.

    d. Calculating peak inspiratory flow during pressure control.

7. During which mode are all breaths the same size?

    a. VC-CMV

    b. PC-CMV

    c. VC-IMV

    d. PC-IMV

    e. PC-CSV

8. Which mode provides full ventilatory support with the highest mean airway pressure for a given tidal volume?

   a. VC-CMV

   b. PC-CMV

   c. VC-IMV

   d. PC-IMV

   e. PC-CSV

9. Pressure Support is an example of which mode?

   a. VC-CMV

   b. PC-CMV

   c. VC-IMV

   d. PC-IMV

   e. PC-CSV

10. Which mode of partial ventilatory support is most often used with neonates?

    a. VC-CMV

    b. PC-CMV

    c. VC-IMV

    d. PC-IMV

    e. PC-CSV

11. Which mode has both volume controlled and pressure controlled breaths?

    a. VC-CMV

    b. PC-CMV

    c. VC-IMV

    d. PC-IMV

    e. PC-CSV

12. Which mode would be most appropriate for a paralyzed patient with unstable lung mechanics?

    a. DC-CMV

   b. PC-CMV

   c. DC-IMV

   d. PC-IMV

   e. DC-CSV

13. Which mode would be most appropriate for a patient with respiratory function who is recovering from anesthesia?

   a. DC-CMV   ___

   b. PC-CMV

   c. DC-IMV

   d. PC-IMV

   e. DC-CSV

14. Suppose you had an awake, alert patient who had an intermittent chest tube leak. Which mode might provide the most stable minute ventilation:

   a. DC-CMV

   b. VC-CMV

   c. VC-IMV

   d. PC-IMV

   e. DC-CSV

Key Ideas

1. From Figure 4-1, what do you have to know in order to calculate inspiratory flow?

2. A recent warning (*Health Devices Alerts* ECRI, August 9, 2002, Vol. 26, No. A32) noted that "...a physician inadvertently increased the tidal volume setting on a Servo 300 ventilator by decreasing the respiratory rate. This problem occurred because the physician was unfamiliar with the ventilator's unique configuration...".   Look at Figure 4-1 and Table 4-1 and explain why tidal volume increased.

3. From Figure 4-4, if tidal volume is held constant, which mode (pressure control or volume control) results in the

highest peak lung pressure? Which produces the highest mean inspiratory pressure? Why?

4. According to Figure 4-5, if the expiratory time is set equal to 3 time constants, how much of the tidal volume will be exhaled before the next breath starts?

5. During pressure controlled ventilation, if inspiratory time is only 2 time constants long, how much of the potential tidal volume will be delivered?

6. If expiratory time is increased from 3 time constants to 5 time constants, how much trapped gas will be avoided?

7. Volutrauma is the result of end inspiratory volume being too large. Explain how this relates to the interaction of tidal volume and PEEP.

ACHTUNG!

Das Machine ist nict fur derfingerpoken und mittengrabben. Ist easy schnappen der Springerwerk, blowenfusen und corkenpoppen mit spitzensparken. Ist nict fur gwrwerken by das Dummkopfen. Das rubbernecken Sightseeren keepen hands in das pockets. Relaxen und watch das Blinkenlights.

Old German folk saying

5. HOW TO READ GRAPHIC DISPLAYS

Rapid Interpretation of Graphic Displays

When learning to read ECGs or radiographic displays, it is useful to look for key features in a specific order. We can apply that technique to waveform displays. The following procedure for routine inspection of ventilator graphics will guide you to look at general features first and then focus on details and potential problems.

1. *Check the overall quality of the display.* Make sure the pressure, volume and flow scales are set correctly and that no portions of the waveforms are cut off. The time scale should be set appropriately; use a fast sweep speed (shorter time scale) if you want to see details of individual breaths and slow sweep (longer time scale) if you want to look at trends. Check to see if leaks (for example, around uncuffed tubes or through chest tubes) are distorting the volume and flow waveforms or preventing an effective determination of static pressure from an inspiratory hold.

2. *Identify the mode of ventilation.* First, try to distinguish between mandatory and spontaneous breaths to determine the breath sequence (such as CMV vs IMV). Then determine if mandatory breaths are volume controlled or pressure controlled. Of course, you could just look at the ventilator to see what mode is set. However, there can be an infinite number of waveform displays for any given mode depending on what the patient is doing, and the whole point is to assess the ventilator-patient interaction. Besides, if the ventilator is not set properly, it may not be delivering the expected mode. For example, if the trigger sensitivity is not set correctly, the patient may be in IMV instead of

SIMV or the pressure support setting may not actually be active.

3. *Check for signs of asynchrony.* From step 2 you should have determined if the patient is making spontaneous breathing efforts. If so, make sure the trigger sensitivity is correctly set. Waveform displays are good for checking how hard the patient must work to trigger a breath and loop displays are good for checking the synchrony between spontaneous and mandatory breaths (particularly useful during infant ventilation). For volume controlled breaths, see if the inspiratory flow is high enough. For pressure controlled breaths, check for proper setting of pressure rise time and cycling threshold (if the ventilator allows such settings). For both types of breaths, determine if there is noticeable gas trapping.

4. *Check for optimal settings and therapeutic response.* This should include an inspection of pressure-volume loops to detect signs of over-distention, indicating a need to reduce tidal volume (this is only reliable for volume controlled breaths). When using an inspiratory hold, you can look at the distance between peak and plateau pressures as an indication of changes in airway resistance (due perhaps to tube kinking or response to bronchodilator). Changes in plateau pressure indicate changes in compliance and may be used to set optimal PEEP levels. Plateau pressure should be below 35 cmH_2O to lessen the risk of lung damage from too large a tidal volume.

You will learn exactly how to look at graphic displays and implement the four step procedure in the rest of this chapter.

Waveform Display Basics

To understand heart physiology we study ECGs and blood pressure waveforms. In the same way, to understand ventilator-patient interaction, we must examine ventilator output waveforms. Ventilator graphics are usually presented in one of two ways. The most common is to plot control variables (pressure, volume, and flow) on the vertical axis and time on the horizontal axis (see Figure 5-1). This type of graphic is often called a **waveform display** (sometimes called a scalar display). The other type of graph plots one control variable against another (such as flow on the vertical axis and volume on the horizontal axis). This is referred to as a **loop display**. We will begin our discussion of output graphics with a detailed description of waveform displays.

Key Idea

> It is important to remember that pressure, volume, and flow are all variables measured relative to their baseline or end-expiratory values. Also, convention dictates that positive flow values (above the horizontal axis) correspond to inspiration, and negative flow values (below the horizontal axis) correspond to expiration. The vertical axes are in units of the measured variables (usually cmH_2O for pressure, liters or mL for volume, and L/minute or L/second for flow). The horizontal axis of these graphs is time, usually in seconds.

Because pressure, volume, and flow are all related by the equation of motion, and because waveform displays are graphs of the variables in the equation of motion, it follows that the shapes of the waveforms are related. To understand this, let's take a closer look at the output waveforms first shown in Chapter 2 (Figure 2-1, redrawn in Figure 5-1 below).

Please note: to simply presentation, the waveforms displayed in this chapter and in most of the rest of the book do not show a PEEP level. Ventilator graphics displays do show PEEP and also the axes labeled in the appropriate units of pressure, volume, flow and time.

Volume Controlled Ventilation

Keep in mind that the equation of motion represents a physical model composed of a rigid flow-conducting tube connected to an elastic chamber (much like a straw connected to a balloon, as shown in Figure 3-1). This physical model represents the airways and the lungs/chest wall. In Figure 5-1, waveforms are plotted for volume controlled ventilation, with constant inspiratory flow, through the airways alone (A), the lungs alone (B), and the two connected (C).

In Figure 5-1A, we see the graph for a model with resistance (the airways) only. A constant flow during inspiration produces a rectangular flow waveform if we include the instantaneous rise at the start of inspiration and the fall back to zero at end inspiration. Volume is the integral of flow (in calculus terms, this is the area between the flow curve and the time axis). For a constant flow, lung volume equals the product of flow and time. Thus, for any inspiratory time, tidal volume equals inspiratory time multiplied by the constant flow. This produces the graph of a straight line with a slope equal to the flow (slope = $\Delta x/\Delta y$, which in this case is change in volume divided by change in time).

Transairway pressure is the product of resistance and flow. Both resistance and flow are constants and the graph of a constant function of time is a straight horizontal line. Another way to look at it is that at each moment, the pressure waveform is just the flow waveform multiplied by the constant resistance, producing the same shape but a different scale. Thus, a rectangular flow waveform produces a rectangular airway pressure waveform. This pressure is the resistive load.

Figure 5-1. Pressure, volume and flow waveforms for different physical models during volume controlled ventilation. A Waveforms for a model with resistance only showing sudden initial rise in pressure at the start of inspiration and then a constant pressure to the end. B Waveforms for a model with elastance only showing a constant rise in pressure from baseline to peak inspiratory pressure. C Waveforms for a model with resistance and elastance, representing the respiratory system. Pressure rises suddenly at the start of inspiration due to resistance and then increases steadily to peak inspiratory pressure due to elastance.

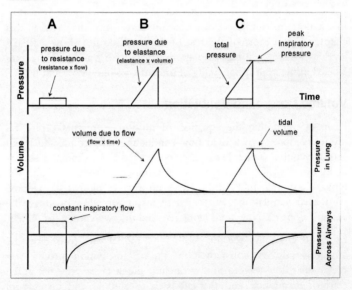

Figure 5-1B shows the results for elastance (the lungs) only. The flow and volume waveforms are of course the same, but the airway pressure waveform is triangular. This is because airway pressure is the product of elastance and volume (a constant and a variable). The result is a graph of a straight line with a slope proportional to the elastance.

Because lung pressure is the product of elastance and volume, lung pressure has the same waveform as volume with just a different vertical scale (with elastance acting like a scaling factor). We called this lung pressure "elastic load" in our earlier discussions.

In Figure 5-1C, we see the waveform for the model of resistance connected in series with elastance (airways and lungs) as it might appear on a ventilator's airway pressure monitor. The flow and volume waveforms are again the same but the airway pressure waveform is the sum of the waveforms in A and B. You can visualize the triangle on top of the rectangle. Another way to look at this is that, for each moment in time, the height of the flow waveform in 5-1C added to the height of the volume waveform in 5-1C equals the height of the pressure waveform in 5-1C.

Predicting the Effects of Changes in Mechanics

Once you understand the above discussion, it will be easy for you to interpret or predict waveform changes associated with changes in respiratory system mechanics. For example, what happens to peak inspiratory pressure if airway resistance increases? Take a minute to figure this out for yourself before you read the answer.

We know that the resistive load is the product of resistance and flow. Thus, if flow stays the same and resistance increases, the resistive load increases and the height of the rectangle in Figure 5-1A would be greater. Thus, the peak pressure in Figure 5-1C would be higher because the triangle sits on a higher rectangle. The same effect would occur if resistance stayed the same and the flow increased.

Here is a little harder question. What happens to peak inspiratory pressure if the patient suddenly gets a massive pneumothorax and one lung collapses? The first thing we have to recognize is that if the remaining lung must accept all the delivered tidal volume, it will take more pressure to expand it. If it takes more pressure to deliver the same volume, then we know that elastance has increased (remember that elastance = Δpressure/Δvolume). In reality, airway resistance may also increase because of the loss of airways, but we will ignore that effect here.

We also know that the elastic load is the product of elastance and volume. Thus, when the patient gets the pneumothorax, the elastic load increases. This is reflected in a higher triangle in Figure 5-1B and a higher peak inspiratory pressure in Figure 5-1C. Also, we said the slope of the inspiratory pressure line is proportional to elastance, so the higher the elastance, the steeper the line.

Now for a really hard question. What happens to mean airway pressure if the patient's compliance improves? First, we have to recall the definitions of mean airway pressure and compliance. Mean airway pressure is proportional to the area under the pressure-time curve for one ventilatory cycle (one inspiration and one expiration).

Extra for Experts

What variables affect mean airway pressure? From Table 4-1, we see that these include (1) the shape of the waveform (such as rectangular versus triangular), (2) the peak inspiratory pressure, (3) end expiratory pressure (PEEP), and (4) the I:E ratio. We know that the flow waveform does not change so the pressure waveform will continue to be triangular. And we are not changing either PEEP or the I:E ratio. That leaves the peak inspiratory pressure. Therefore, we have to determine the effect of increasing compliance on peak inspiratory pressure.

Recall that the definition of compliance is tidal volume divided by the difference between peak inspiratory pressure and PEEP. Thus, if compliance increases and PEEP is unchanged, peak pressure must decrease.

If peak pressure decreases, the area under the triangle in Figure 5-1B decreases and the area under the total airway pressure waveform in Figure 5-1C will decrease. This leads to the conclusion that if compliance increases, mean airway pressure decreases.

The results of these analyses are shown in Figure 5-2.

The examples given above are not just intellectual exercises. The ability to make accurate explanations and predictions, based on theoretical relationships, is what distinguishes an expert in mechanical ventilation. A novice can set up a mechanical ventilator and make setting changes in response to the patient's needs. But a novice seldom considers how one pattern of settings (or mode) might compare to an alternative pattern. And when he does have some understanding, he can rarely explain it clearly and consistently to others. An expert knows what to expect before it happens and can describe in detail the meaning of the observed patterns of pressure, volume and flow in terms of both mechanics and physiology. One of the goals of this book is to help the reader to advance to the expert level.

Figure 5-2. Effects of changing respiratory system mechanics on airway pressure during volume controlled ventilation. Dashed line shows original waveform before the change A Increased resistance causes an increase in the initial pressure at the start of inspiration and a higher peak inspiratory pressure and higher mean pressure. B An increase in elastance (decrease in compliance) causes no change in initial pressure but a higher peak inspiratory pressure and higher mean pressure. C A decrease in elastance (increase in compliance) causes no change in initial pressure but a lower peak inspiratory pressure and lower mean pressure.

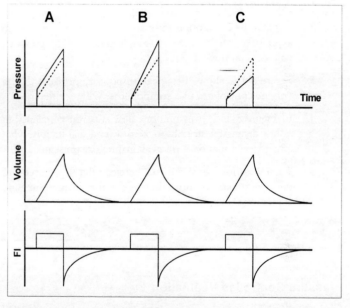

While we are on the subject of mean airway pressure, what happens if ventilatory frequency is increased? From Table 4-1 again we see that of the four variables that determine mean airway pressure, frequency is not mentioned. But from Figures 4-1, 4-3 and Table 4-1 we see that frequency is related to I:E ratio. Frequency can be increased while I:E is held constant (by decreasing both T_I and T_E) in which case mean airway pressure is unchanged. Alternatively, if frequency is altered by changing I:E, then mean airway changes in the same direction as I:E. For example, increasing frequency by decreasing expiratory time increases the I:E ratio and increases mean airway pressure.

Mechanical Ventilation

The analyses above were for volume controlled ventilation with a constant inspiratory flow. Similar analyses can be applied to volume controlled ventilation with other flow waveforms and to pressure controlled ventilation. Take another look at Figure 4-4. Perhaps now you can better appreciate the use of shading and the dashed lines indicating mean airway pressure.

Review and Consider

1. Describe the four-step procedure for routine inspection of ventilator graphics.

2. Explain the convention for distinguishing inspiration from expiration on waveform graphics showing pressure, volume, and flow versus time.

3. Figure 5-1 C shows that peak inspiratory pressure during volume control has two components. What are they?

4. In Figure 5-1 C, if inspiratory flow was not constant but rather decreased steadily to zero at end inspiration, what effect would that have on peak inspiratory pressure?

5. What does it mean if the area between the flow curve and the time axis is not the same for inspiration and expiration?

Pressure Controlled Ventilation

In Figure 5-3, waveforms are plotted for pressure controlled ventilation, with constant inspiratory pressure. As we break out the components of the waveform for models of the airways alone, and the lungs alone, as we did in Figure 5-1, we will assume that inspiratory flow retains the decaying exponential waveform for the purposes of the illustration (which it would not do if you actually hooked up a model of resistance only to a ventilator in a pressure controlled mode).

Figure 5- 3. Pressure, volume and flow waveforms for different physical models during pressure controlled ventilation. A Waveforms for a model with resistance only. B Waveforms for a model with elastance only. C Waveforms for a model with resistance and elastance, representing the respiratory system. Note that like Figure 5-1, the height of the pressure waveform at each moment is determined by the height of the flow waveform added to the height of the volume waveform.

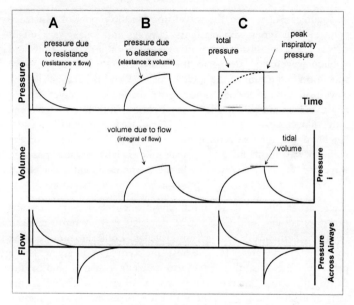

In Figure 5-3A, we see the graph for a model with resistance (the airways) only. The exponential flow during inspiration starts instantaneously at peak inspiratory flow and decreases to zero at end inspiration. Volume is the integral of flow (in calculus terms, this is the area between the flow curve and the time axis). For an exponential flow, lung volume is also exponential starting at zero and rising asymptotically[1] to the tidal volume (see Table 4-1).

Transairway pressure is the product of resistance and flow. The pressure waveform (the resistive load) is just the flow waveform multiplied by the constant resistance, producing the same shape as flow but a different scale. Thus, an exponential flow waveform produces an exponential airway pressure waveform.

---

[1] An asymptote is a curve that continually approaches nearer to some value but though infinitely extended, would never meet it.

Figure 5-3B, shows the results for elastance (the lungs) only. The flow and volume waveforms are of course the same, but the airway pressure waveform (the elastic load) is exponential. This is because airway pressure is the product of elastance and volume (a constant and a variable). Just like with resistance and flow, elastance, being constant, acts like a scaling factor for the pressure waveform, preserving the shape of the volume waveform.

In Figure 5-3C, we see the waveform for the model of resistance connected in series with elastance (airways and lungs) as it might appear on a ventilator's airway pressure monitor. The flow and volume waveforms are again the same, but the airway pressure waveform is the sum of the waveforms in A and B. Graphically, the waveform for elastic load is the same shape as the waveform for resistive load turned upside down because both curves have the same time constant. As in Figure 5-1C, for each moment in time, the height of the flow waveform in 5-1C added to the height of the volume waveform in 5-1C equals the height of the pressure waveform in 5-1C. When you add the falling exponential waveform to its mirror image (a rising exponential) you get a straight line.

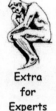

There is another way to think about the relationship between pressure, volume, and flow waveforms that may be more relevant both mathematically and physiologically. Look at the pressure waveform in Figure 5-1C. Because the ventilator is acting like a pressure controller, this waveform remains constant and is the driving force that generates the flow and volume waveforms. At the start of inspiration (t = 0), the ventilator forces the airway pressure to suddenly rise above baseline to the pressure limit. At that moment, pressure at the airway opening is, say, 25 cm H_2O. But pressure in the lungs is still at baseline, or 25 cm H_2O less than the airway opening. This pressure differential causes an instantaneous rise in flow. From Table 4-1 we see that

$$\dot{V}_I = \left(\frac{\Delta P}{R}\right)\left(e^{-t/\tau}\right) = \left(\frac{\Delta P}{R}\right)\left(e^{-0/\tau}\right) = \left(\frac{\Delta P}{R}\right)\left(e^0\right) = \left(\frac{\Delta P}{R}\right)(1) = \left(\frac{\Delta P}{R}\right)$$

which shows that the instant inspiration starts, flow is at its highest value equal to the pressure gradient divided by resistance.

Also at this moment, even though flow is some positive number, volume is zero because time is still zero. To verify this we look at the equation for volume from Table 4-1:

$$V_T = \Delta P \times C \times \left(1 - e^{-t/\tau}\right)$$

where ΔP is 25 cm H_2O, C and τ can be any value. When inspiratory time $(t) = 0$, the $-t/\tau = 0/\tau = 0$, the expression $e^{-t/\tau} = e^0 = 1$, the expression $(1 - e^{-t/\tau}) = (1 - 1) = 0$, and thus $V_T = 25 \times C \times 0 = 0$.

At each moment in time, the driving force causing flow (airway pressure minus lung pressure) gets smaller because airway pressure is controlled at a constant value but lung pressure increases as volume accumulates. It is this continuous decrease in driving pressure that results in the characteristic exponential waveforms for flow and volume.

As inspiration progresses, tidal volume increases until, at inspiratory time = infinity, it reaches a maximum value equal to $\Delta P \times C$. Of course, tidal volume gets very close to this maximum value much sooner. The symbol τ is the time constant. Recall from our earlier discussion about time constants that when the inspiratory time equals $3 \times \tau$ tidal volume will be 95% of its maximum value (see Figure 4-5).

Predicting the Effects of Changes in Mechanics

Now let's predict waveform changes associated with changes in respiratory system mechanics, just as we did for volume controlled ventilation. For example, what happens to peak inspiratory pressure if airway resistance increases?

This is really a trick question. Pressure controlled ventilation, by definition, implies that the airway pressure waveform stays constant (including its shape, peak value and mean value) regardless of changes in respiratory system mechanics (see Figure 3-2).

OK, so what happens to tidal volume if airway resistance increases? You could approach this question mathematically and just inspect the equation for volume during pressure controlled ventilation from Table 4-1. The equation would tell us that the time constant is increased, so it takes longer for a given volume to accumulate. But since the inspiratory time remains the same, there is not enough time to accumulate as much volume, so the tidal volume decreases.

There is a more intuitive approach to this question involving waveforms. First, consider what happens to peak inspiratory flow when resistance increases. Because peak flow is equal to $\Delta P/R$, as resistance increases, peak flow decreases. Now look at Figure 5-3 and see that if ~~peak~~ flow decreases, the area under the flow waveform has to decrease. Because tidal volume is proportional to the area under the flow waveform (the integral of flow with respect to time) then when resistance increases, tidal volume decreases.

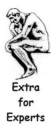

**Extra
for
Experts**

Here is a little harder question. What happens to tidal volume if the patient suddenly gets a massive pneumothorax and one lung collapses? First, we must recognize that a collapsed lung will result in a decrease in respiratory system compliance. How do we know this? We said before that the lungs can be modeled as two compliances connected in parallel and compliances in parallel add like resistors in series (they simply add together). Therefore, removing one compliant component (collapsing one lung) decreases the total compliance. The equation for tidal volume during pressure controlled ventilation is:

$$V_T = \Delta P \times C \times \left(1 - e^{-t/\tau}\right)$$

The parameters in this equation that are affected by the pneumothorax are compliance, C and the time constant, τ. Decreasing compliance decreases the maximum tidal volume, which is compliance times ΔP (the change in airway pressure above baseline, or PIP-PEEP). Decreasing compliance also decreases the time constant, so ~~that~~ more of the maximum volume will accumulate each moment. These two effects seem to work against each other and it is hard to imagine which will have the greater effect. One way to find out is to program the equation into a computer spreadsheet and try different values of compliance and inspiratory time. If you do that, you will find that the effect of changing compliance is larger than that of changing the time constant, so as compliance decreases, tidal volume also decreases.

The results of these analyses are shown in Figure 5-4.

While we are on the subject, I would suggest that you experiment with all the equations given in this book, either with a computer or graphing calculator. That way you will be able to generate your own illustrations (like Figures 5-3 and 5-4) and verify your theoretical conclusions. You cannot attain expert level in mechanical ventilation until you have some experience doing this.

Figure 5-4. Effects of changing respiratory system mechanics on airway pressure during pressure controlled ventilation. A Waveforms before any changes. B Increased resistance causes a decrease in peak inspiratory flow, a lower tidal volume, and a longer time constant. Note that inspiration is time cycled before flow decays to zero. C An increase in elastance (decrease in compliance) causes no change in peak inspiratory flow but decreases tidal volume and decreases the time constant.

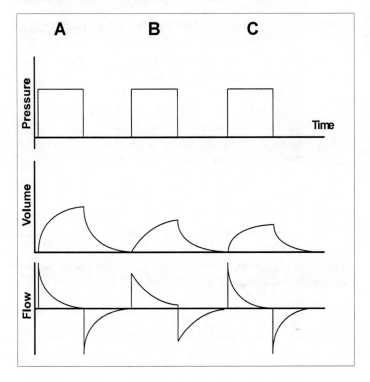

Notice that in Figures 5-1 and 5-3, all the expiratory flow waveforms are the same. From Table 4-1 we see that passive expiration is governed by the equation:

$$\dot{V}_E = -\left(\frac{\Delta P}{R}\right)\left(e^{-t/\tau}\right)$$

Because ΔP is the tidal volume divided by compliance, and because the tidal volume and compliance and time constants are assumed to be the same in all the models, the flow curves must be the same

- 133 -

shape. Peak expiratory flow happens at time = 0 (the start of expiration). If you substitute 0 for t in the above equation you see that peak expiratory flow is $-\Delta P / R$. This is the same result for peak inspiratory flow during pressure controlled ventilation with a rectangular pressure waveform, except that inspiratory flow is positive rather than negative.

Review and Consider

6. What is the difference between assisted ventilation with a constant inspiratory pressure and ventilation with a rectangular pressure waveform?

7. Look at Figure 5-3 C. What do you think would happen to the shape of the pressure waveform if you adjusted the pressure rise on the ventilator so that it took longer to reach the pressure limit? What would be the effect on peak inspiratory flow?

8. During pressure controlled ventilation what value for inspiratory time will give the largest tidal volume?

9. For passive expiration, flow decays asymptotically. When does it reach zero?

Volume Controlled vs. Pressure Controlled Ventilation

Now that you are familiar with the waveforms associated with volume and pressure controlled ventilation, let's try to predict what will happen if we switch a patient from one mode to the other. The newer, more advanced modes of ventilation are available on all top-of-the-line ICU ventilators. Yet it seems that volume controlled IMV remains the most commonly used mode. Many patients start in this mode and stay there unless their condition seriously deteriorates. Then clinicians start to think about switching to pressure control. Frequently, they will say that they are interested in decreasing the patient's risk of volutrauma by using lower peak inspiratory pressure or that pressure control seems to improve oxygenation. A closer look at the waveforms for these two modes may help to understand what is really going on.

Figure 5-5 is another comparison of waveforms for volume control and pressure control. To make the comparison fair, the tidal volume has been made the same for each. Looking at the pressure waveforms, we notice a striking difference in peak inspiratory pressures. This is what some clinicians feel is a benefit. But it may be a misconception.

Figure 5-5. Volume control compared to pressure control at the same tidal volume. On the pressure waveforms the dotted lines show that peak inspiratory pressure is higher for volume control. On the volume/lung pressure waveforms, the dotted lines show (a) peak lung pressure is the same for both modes and (b) that pressure control results in a larger volume at mid inspiration.

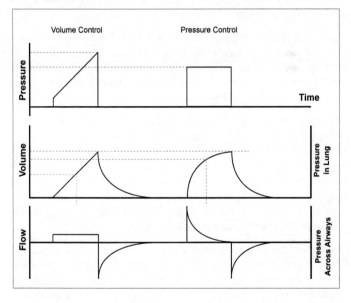

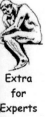

The lungs may be damaged by over-expansion, which correlates with high peak transalveolar pressures. However, transalveolar pressure is not very well predicted by the inspiratory pressure displayed on the ventilator (transrespiratory pressure). This is because transrespiratory pressure is the sum of transairway pressure and transthoracic pressure. Transairway pressure is due to flow and resistance. Thus, an elevated peak inspiratory pressure may be due simply to a change in flow or resistance and have nothing to do with lung expansion. Transthoracic pressure is composed of transalveolar pressure and transmural pressure. This means that inspiratory pressure could be elevated because of a stiff chest wall, which would tend to protect the lungs from over-expansion.

To summarize, the inspiratory pressure displayed on the ventilator is a poor predictor of the transalveolar pressure that may cause lung damage because there are so many other variables in between:

$$P_{TR} = P_{TA} + P_{TT} = P_{TAry} + (P_{TAlv} + P_{TM})$$

where P_{TR} is the transrespiratory pressure displayed on the ventilator's airway pressure display, P_{TAry} is transairway pressure due to flow and resistance, P_{TT} is transthoracic pressure, P_{TAlv} is transalveolar pressure due to volume and lung compliance, P_{TM} is transmural pressure due to volume and chest wall compliance.

Figure 5-5 shows that the pressure controlled breath has a lower peak inspiratory pressure than the volume controlled breath. Looking at the volume curves, we see that because both breaths have the same tidal volume, *they both result in the same lung pressure and presumably the same risk of lung damage.*

As we discussed before, the reason that pressure control has a lower peak inspiratory pressure at the airway opening is that it has a very different flow waveform. It starts out with a high flow and high transairway pressure (flow times resistance) at a time when lung volume and lung pressure are zero. Then as lung pressure increases, inspiratory flow and transairway pressure drop exponentially. At end inspiration they are nearly zero. Most of the transrespiratory pressure at that time is due to lung pressure.

In contrast, the volume controlled breath has a constant inspiratory flow and thus constant transairway pressure throughout inspiration. At end inspiration, there is a substantially larger component of transrespiratory pressure due to resistance. We can unmask this effect by creating an inspiratory hold and observing the static (no flow) pressure as shown in Figure 5-6. Now, the transrespiratory pressure at end inspiration is due entirely to the elastic recoil of the lungs. This static pressure is often called **plateau pressure**. We can use plateau pressure to calculate both the static compliance of the lungs and inspiratory airway resistance. Plateau pressure is achieved with an inspiratory hold during volume controlled ventilation or with a sufficiently long inspiratory time (to attain zero flow at end inspiration) during pressure controlled ventilation.

$$compliance = \frac{tidal\ volume}{plateau\ pressure - baseline\ pressure}$$

$$resistance = \frac{peak\ inspiratory\ pressure - baseline\ pressure}{inspiratory\ flow}$$

where baseline pressure is the PEEP or CPAP setting on the ventilator. These equations can be used to estimate compliance and resistance by hand from readings you take from the ventilator display. When the ventilator calculates these parameters, it usually measures pressure, volume, and flow every few milliseconds and fits the equation of motion to the data set using linear regression. However, some ventilators will calculate static compliance using an inspiratory hold and the equation above.

Figure 5-6. Waveforms associated with an inspiratory hold during volume controlled ventilation. Notice that inspiratory flow time is less than inspiratory time and flow goes to zero during the inspiratory pause time while pressure drops from peak to plateau.

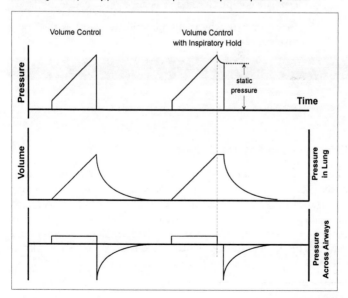

Look again at Figure 5-5. Can we say something about why oxygenation might be better with pressure control? The dotted lines on the volume curves mark the volume accumulated at about half way through inspiration. Notice that the lung volume at this time is greater for pressure control. The flow waveform for pressure control results in expansion of the lungs earlier in inspiration and hence allows more time for gas exchange to occur. It also results in a higher mean airway pressure, as evidenced by the larger area under the volume/lung pressure curve (in fact you could fit the volume control curve inside the pressure control curve). These effects can definitely improve oxygenation in some patients.

Review and Consider

10. Explain why current guidelines[2] for lung protective strategies suggest keeping plateau pressure, rather than peak inspiratory pressure, below 30 cmH$_2$O.

11. Explain how pressure controlled ventilation might result in better oxygenation than volume controlled ventilation.

12. What measurements do you have to make in order to estimate compliance and resistance at the bedside?

13. In Figure 5-6, why is the plateau pressure less than peak inspiratory pressure?

Effects of the Patient Circuit

The pressure, volume, and flow the patient actually receives are never precisely the same as what the clinician sets on the ventilator. Sometimes these differences are caused by instrument inaccuracies or calibration error. More commonly, the patient delivery circuit contributes to discrepancies between the desired and actual patient values. This is because the patient circuit has its own compliance

---

[2] Respir Care2001:46(10)1024-1037.

and resistance. Thus, the pressure measured on the inspiratory side of a ventilator will always be higher than the pressure at the airway opening due to patient circuit resistance. In addition, the volume and flow coming out of the ventilator will exceed that delivered to the patient because of the compliance of the patient circuit.

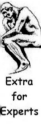

Extra for Experts

Exactly how the mechanical properties of the patient circuit affect ventilator performance depends on whether they are connected in series or in parallel with the patient. It turns out that the resistance of the patient circuit is connected in series while the compliance is modeled as a parallel connection. To understand this, we first make the simplifying assumption that we can examine the patient circuit's resistance separate from its compliance. It is intuitively obvious that the same flow of gas that comes from the ventilator travels through the circuit tubing as through the patient's airway opening. We can also see that the pressure drop across the patient circuit will be different from that across the respiratory system because they have different resistances. Recall from Chapter 3 that when two circuit components share the same flow but have different pressure drops, they are connected in series. This means that the patient circuit resistance, however small, adds to the total resistive load seen by the ventilator. Thus, in a volume controlled breath the peak inspiratory pressure is higher and in a pressure controlled breath, the tidal volume and peak flow are lower. In practice, the effect of the patient circuit resistance is usually ignored because it is so much lower than the resistance of the respiratory system.

Now consider the patient circuit compliance.[3] As the ventilator delivers the breath to the patient, pressure at the airway opening rises relative to atmospheric pressure, which is the driving force for flow into the lungs. The patient circuit is connected between the ventilator and the airway, so the pressure it experiences across its walls is the same as that experienced by the respiratory system (remember we are ignoring its resistance now so we can ignore any pressure drop between the ventilator outlet and the airway opening). The volume change of the patient circuit tubing will be different from that of the respiratory system because the compliance of the circuit is different. Because the patient circuit and the respiratory system fill with different volumes during the same inspiratory time, the flows they experience are different (remember that flow =

---

[3] The effective compliance of the patient circuit is a combination of the tubing compliance and the compressibility of the gas inside it.

volume ÷ time). Again, from Chapter 3 if two circuit components share the same pressure drop but different flows, they are connected in parallel. Because they are in parallel, the two compliances are additive, so the total compliance is greater than either component.

Patient circuit compliance can sometimes be greater than respiratory system compliance and thus have a large effect on ventilation. It must be accounted for either automatically by the ventilator or by manually increasing the tidal volume. For example, when ventilating neonates, the patient circuit compliance can be as much as three times that of the respiratory system, even with small-bore tubing and a small volume humidifier. Thus, when trying to deliver a preset tidal volume during volume controlled ventilation, as little as 25% of the set volume will be delivered to the patient with 75% compressed in the patient circuit. The compliance of the patient circuit can be determined by occluding the tubing at the patient wye, delivering a small volume under flow control (using zero PEEP), and noting the resulting pressure. Using a short inspiratory hold will make it easier to read the pressure. Then compliance is calculated as before by dividing the volume by the pressure. Once the patient circuit compliance is known, the set tidal volume can be corrected using the following equation:

$$V_{delivered} = \frac{V_{set}}{1 + \dfrac{C_{PC}}{C_{RS}}}$$

where $V_{delivered}$ is the tidal volume delivered to the patient, V_{set} is the tidal volume setting on the ventilator, C_{PC} is the patient circuit compliance, and C_{RS} is the respiratory system compliance. We can get a more intuitive understanding of this equation if we put in some values. Suppose, for example, that we use the perfect patient circuit that has zero compliance. Substituting zero for C_{PC} we get

$$V_{delivered} = \frac{V_{set}}{1 + \dfrac{C_{PC}}{C_{RS}}} = \frac{V_{set}}{1 + \dfrac{0}{C_{RS}}} = \frac{V_{set}}{1 + 0} = \frac{V_{set}}{1} = V_{set}$$

which shows that there is no effect on the delivered tidal volume. Suppose now that C_{PC} is as large as C_{RS} ($C_{PC} = C_{RS}$). Now we have:

$$V_{delivered} = \frac{V_{set}}{1 + \dfrac{C_{PC}}{C_{RS}}} = \frac{V_{set}}{1 + 1} = \frac{V_{set}}{2}$$

in which case half of the volume from the ventilator goes to the patient and the other half is compressed in the patient circuit.

The effect of the patient circuit is more troublesome during volume controlled modes than pressure controlled modes. This is because during volume control, the ventilator meters out a specific volume of gas and unless it measures flow at the airway opening, it has no way of knowing how much goes to the patient and how much goes to the patient circuit. In contrast, during pressure controlled modes the ventilator simply meters out a set pressure change no matter where the gas goes. Because the respiratory system and the patient circuit compliance are in parallel, they both experience the same driving pressure (peak inspiratory pressure minus end expiratory pressure) so tidal volume delivery is affected very little. The only effect might be that the patient circuit compliance may tend to increase the pressure rise time which would tend to decrease peak flow and tidal volume slightly.

Another area where patient circuit compliance causes trouble is in the determination of autoPEEP. One method to determine autoPEEP during mechanical ventilation is to manually create an expiratory hold (delay the next inspiration) until static conditions prevail throughout the lungs (no flow anywhere in the lungs). The pressure at this time (total PEEP) minus the applied PEEP is autoPEEP. AutoPEEP ($PEEP_A$) is an index of the gas trapped in the system at end expiration due to an insufficient expiratory time:

$$measured\ PEEP_A = \frac{V_{trapped}}{C_{total}}$$

where $PEEP_A$ is autoPEEP, $V_{trapped}$ is the volume of gas trapped in the patient and the patient circuit at end expiration (above that associated with applied PEEP) and C_{total} is the total compliance of the respiratory system and the patient circuit. The problem is that we want autoPEEP to reflect the gas trapped in the patient, not in the circuit. If we know the compliances of the patient circuit and the respiratory system, we can correct the measured autoPEEP as follows:

$$true\,PEEP_A = \frac{C_{RS} + C_{PC}}{C_{RS}} \times measured\,PEEP_A$$

where true $PEEP_A$ is the autoPEEP in the lungs, measured $PEEP_A$ is the autoPEEP in the lungs and patient circuit, C_{RS} is the respiratory system compliance, and C_{PC} is the patient circuit compliance. If the ventilator displays autoPEEP on its monitor, check the ventilator operator's manual to see whether or not the autoPEEP calculation is corrected for patient circuit compliance. The larger C_{PC} is relative to C_{RS}, the larger the error will be. Again, the error will be most noticeable in pediatric and neonatal patients.

Review and Consider

14. Explain, in terms of circuit compliance and resistance, what happens if you try to ventilate a neonate with pediatric sized patient circuit.

15. What happens if you try to ventilate an adult with a pediatric sized circuit?

Idealized Waveform Displays

Many ventilators have monitors that display pressure, volume, and flow waveforms providing the clinician with information to evaluate ventilator-patient interaction. However, many confounding variables can affect the way waveforms look. Leaks in the system, condensation in the patient circuit, inaccuracies in the ventilator flow and pressure control system and effects of the patient's respiratory system mechanics or ventilatory efforts can all create distorted waveforms. For this reason, it is important for you to know what theoretical or "ideal" waveforms should look like, so that you can then recognize when something is wrong. Such graphs can also help you to appreciate how different control variable waveforms affect mean airway pressure.

Figure 5-7 illustrates some of the most common ventilator output waveforms. These waveforms were in fact generated with a computer. They are graphs of the equation of motion for various types of waveform settings.

The waveforms were created as follows:

1. Define the control waveform mathematically. For example, an ascending ramp flow waveform is specified as *flow = constant x time*.

2. Set the tidal volume to equal 644 mL (equivalent to about 9 mL/kg for an adult).

3. Specify the desired values for airway resistance (20 cmH$_2$O/L/s) and respiratory system compliance (20 mL/ cmH$_2$O) according to American National Standards Institute recommendations.

4. Substitute the above data into the equation of motion and solve for the unknown variables. For example, if we input the equation for flow, we solve for volume and pressure.

5. Plot the resulting equations for pressure, volume, and flow as functions of time.

Figure 5-7. Theoretical pressure, volume, and flow waveforms for the same tidal volume and inspiratory time. (A) pressure control with a rectangular pressure waveform; (B) flow control with a rectangular flow waveform; (C) flow control with an ascending ramp flow waveform; (D) flow control with a descending ramp flow waveform; (E) flow control with a sinusoidal flow waveform. Short dashed lines represent mean inspiratory pressure. Long dashed lines show mean airway pressure.

Key Idea

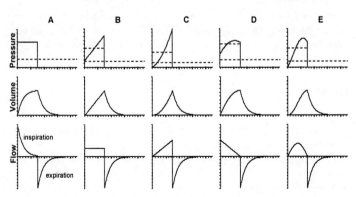

Because the waveforms in Figure 5-7 are generated by mathematical models (as graphs of the equation of motion), they do not show the minor deviations or "noise" often seen during actual ventilator use. Such noise can be caused by many factors, including vibration and turbulence (e.g., from condensation in the patient circuit). These waveforms also do not show the effect of expiratory circuit resistance because this varies depending on the ventilator and type of circuit. Nor do the waveforms show the various indicators of problems with ventilator-patient synchrony (e.g., improper sensitivity setting, and gas trapping), which will be discussed later. Lastly, one must remember that waveform appearances change when the time scale is altered. A faster sweep (shorter time scale) will tend to widen a given waveform, while a slower sweep speed (longer time scale) will show many waveforms together on the screen.

Most ventilator waveforms are either rectangular, exponential, ramp, or sinusoidal in shape.[4] Although a variety of subtypes is possible, we will describe only the most common. Waveforms are listed according to the shape of the control variable waveform. Any new waveforms produced by future ventilators can easily be accommodated by this system.

Pressure

Rectangular

Mathematically, a rectangular waveform is referred to as a step (instantaneous) change in transrespiratory pressure from one value to another (Figure 5-6, *A*). In response, volume rises exponentially from zero to a steady state value equal to compliance times the change in airway pressure (that is, PIP-PEEP). Inspiratory flow falls exponentially from a peak value (at the start of inspiration) equal to (PIP-PEEP) divided by resistance.

Exponential

Exponential pressure waveforms can be produced by adjusting the pressure rise control on some newer intensive care ventilators. The resulting pressure and volume waveforms can take on a variety of shapes ranging from an exponential rise (same shape as the volume

---

[4] Respir Care 1991;36:347-356.

waveform in Figure 5-7, *A*) to a linear rise (same shape as the volume waveform in Figure 5-7, *B*). In general, the flow waveform is similar to that seen in Figure 5-7, *A*, except that peak inspiratory flow is reached gradually rather than instantaneously (resulting in a rounded rather than peaked waveform), and peak flow is lower than with a rectangular pressure waveform. In response, the volume waveform initially rises very slowly, then at peak flow, rises rapidly in an exponential fashion.

Sinusoidal

A sinusoidal pressure waveform can be created by attaching a piston to a rotating crank. In addition, a linear drive motor driven by a microprocessor can produce a sine wave pressure pattern. In response, the volume and flow waveforms are also sinusoidal but they attain their peak values at different times (Figure 5-7, *E*).

Oscillating

Oscillating pressure waveforms can take on a variety of shapes, from sinusoidal to ramp (SensorMedics 3100 Oscillator), to roughly triangular (Infrasonics Star Oscillator). The distinguishing feature of a ventilator classified as an oscillator is that it can generate negative transrespiratory pressure. That is, if the mean airway pressure is set equal to atmospheric pressure, then the airway pressure waveform oscillates above and below zero.

If the pressure waveform is sinusoidal, volume and flow will also be sinusoidal but out of phase with each other (that is, their peak values occur at different times).

Volume

Ramp

Volume controllers that produce an ascending ramp waveform produce a linear rise in volume from zero at the start of inspiration to the peak value, or set tidal volume, at end-inspiration (Figure 5-7, *B*). In response, the flow waveform is rectangular. The pressure waveform rises instantaneously from zero to a value equal to (resistance times flow) at the start of inspiration. From here, it rises linearly to its peak value (PIP) equal to (tidal volume x elastance) + (flow x resistance).

Sinusoidal

This volume waveform is most often produced by ventilators whose drive mechanism is a piston attached to a rotating crank (such as Emerson ventilators). The output waveform of this type of ventilator can be approximated by the first half of a cosine curve, whose shape in this case is referred to as a sigmoidal curve (Figure 5-7, *E*). Because volume is sinusoidal during inspiration, pressure and flow are also sinusoidal.

Flow

Rectangular

A rectangular flow waveform is perhaps the most common output (Figure 5-7, *B*). When the flow waveform is rectangular, volume is a ramp waveform and pressure is a step followed by a ramp as described for the ramp volume waveform.

Ramp

Many respiratory care practitioners and ventilator manufacturers refer to ramp waveforms (and sometimes exponential waveforms) as either "accelerating" or "decelerating" flow patterns. But the use of these terms is usually inappropriate. If a car slows, we do not say that its velocity decelerates; we say that the *car* decelerates. We do not say that a cyclotron is a velocity accelerator but that it is a *particle* accelerator. The rate of change of position of an object is the velocity of the object; analogously, the rate of change of volume is flow. The rate of change of velocity of an object is the acceleration of the object; likewise, the rate of change of flow is the acceleration of volume, *not* the acceleration of flow. Therefore, if we want to say that flow changes, we should simply talk about an increasing flow or a decreasing flow (or an accelerating volume or a decelerating volume), *not* an accelerating flow or a decelerating flow.

Ascending Ramp

A true ascending ramp waveform starts at zero and increases linearly to the peak value (Figure 5-7, *C*). Ventilator flow waveforms are usually truncated. Inspiration starts with an initial instantaneous flow (for example, the Bear-5 starts inspiration at 50% of the set peak flow). Flow then increases linearly to the set peak flow rate. In response to an ascending ramp flow waveform, the pressure and volume waveforms are exponential with a concave upward shape.

Descending Ramp

A true descending ramp waveform starts at the peak value and decreases linearly to zero (Figure 5-7, *D*). Ventilator flow waveforms are usually truncated; inspiratory flow rate decreases linearly from the set peak flow until it reaches some arbitrary threshold where flow drops immediately to zero (for example, the Puritan Bennett 7200a ends inspiration when the flow rate drops to 5 L/min). In response to a descending ramp flow waveform, the pressure and volume waveforms are exponential with a concave downward shape.

Sinusoidal

Some ventilators offer a mode in which the inspiratory flow waveform approximates the shape of the first half of a sine wave (Figure 5-7, *E*). As with the ramp waveform, ventilators often truncate the sine waveform by starting and ending flow at some percentage of the set peak flow rather than start and end at zero flow. In response to a sinusoidal flow waveform, the pressure and volume waveforms will also be sinusoidal but out of phase with each other.

Recognizing Modes

As with the previous discussion of control variable waveforms, we will continue to use idealized waveforms. This will give us some frame of reference when we try to identify problems later. The one difference in the following waveforms is that the imaginary muscle pressure has been added as the top graph. This will help us to appreciate the nature of the ventilator-patient interaction. Although we don't measure muscle pressure directly, and ventilator graphics cannot show it, we can draw arbitrarily shaped curves that indicate the presence and strength of the patient's breathing efforts. Muscle pressure is effectively a positive change in transrespiratory pressure, just like ventilator pressure, and is thus shown going above the time axis.

One thing to keep in mind is that the waveforms that follow are all "idealized". They do not show the irregularities that you will see on real ventilator monitors. Real waveforms are often very "noisy" or jagged in appearance. Their relative shapes will also be different for various specific ventilator settings (peak flow, pressure, tidal volume, etc). Anther major difference is that the compliance of the patient circuit tends to round all the sharp corners. It would be impractical to illustrate the many possible shapes of even one particular mode of ventilation. What you need to learn here is the general shape of the waveforms for each mode of ventilation and to pick out the major characteristics. This will help you to identify a mode at a glance and to focus on any particular problems.

16. During VC-CMV, you change from constant flow to a descending ramp waveform. What do you expect to happen to peak inspiratory pressure and mean airway pressure?

17. The short dashed lines in Figure 5-7 represent mean inspiratory pressure. Why is mean inspiratory pressure higher than mean airway pressure? Why is there no mean inspiratory pressure line for A?

18. What is meant by the term "decelerating" flow?

Continuous Mandatory Ventilation (CMV)

VC-CMV

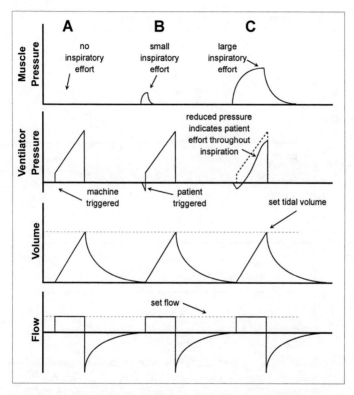

Breaths during volume controlled continuous mandatory ventilation can be machine triggered (A) or patient triggered (B). Although VC-CMV is often chosen to rest the patient, patient effort does not necessarily stop. The area of the pressure curve *under* the baseline is proportional to the work the patient does on the ventilator (imposed work). The area under the pressure curve *above* the baseline is the work the ventilator does on the patient. The difference in the areas between passive inspiration (A) and active inspiration (C) is proportional to the work the patient does during inspiration.

PC-CMV(rectangular pressure waveform)

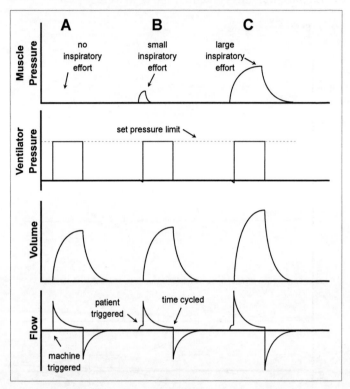

This figure shows pressure control ventilation with an idealized rectangular pressure waveform. Breaths during pressure controlled continuous mandatory ventilation can be machine triggered (A) or patient triggered (B). This figure illustrates flow triggering as opposed to pressure triggering shown for VC-CMV. Notice that in contrast to volume control, in pressure control, large patient efforts (C) do not affect the pressure waveform but do affect flow and volume.

PC-IMV (exponential pressure waveform)

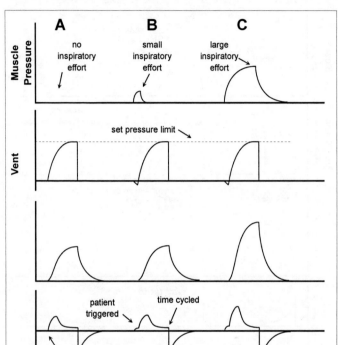

Few ventilators actually generate a rectangular pressure waveform as shown in the previous figure. More often, you see an exponential rise at the beginning of the airway pressure curve. This applies to all forms of pressure control (except Proportional Assist) and dual control between breaths. If the pressure rise time is adjustable, and the rise time is increased, the pressure waveform changes from more rectangular (see previous figure) to more exponential as shown above. Note that when the pressure waveform is changed from rectangular to exponential, the flow waveform changes and peak inspiratory flow decreases.

Mechanical Ventilation

DC-CMV (dual control between breaths)

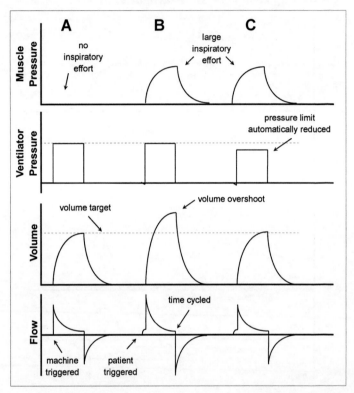

Dual control between breaths will automatically compensate for changes in mechanics or patient effort over the course of several breaths. During steady-state, the pressure limit is just high enough to achieve the set tidal volume (A). If the patient suddenly makes a large inspiratory effort, muscle pressure adds to ventilator pressure and the resultant tidal volume is larger than the set value (B). The ventilator compensates by lowering the pressure limit (C).

DC-CMV (dual control within breaths: pressure control to volume control)

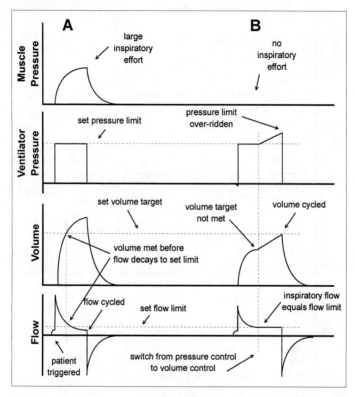

In (A) the patient's inspiratory effort is assisted by a Pressure Support type breath. The tidal volume target is met before flow decays to the set flow limit, and the breath is flow cycled. If the patient effort decreases enough that tidal volume is not met by the time flow decays to the set flow limit, then the control variable switches from pressure to volume (B). The breath proceeds at the set flow limit and is volume cycled when the target tidal volume is met. Notice that when this happens, airway pressure rises above the set pressure limit. Examples of this mode are Volume Assured Pressure Support on the Bird 8400 and Tbird ventilators and Pressure Augment on the Bear 1000 ventilator.

DC-CMV (dual control within breaths: volume control to pressure control)

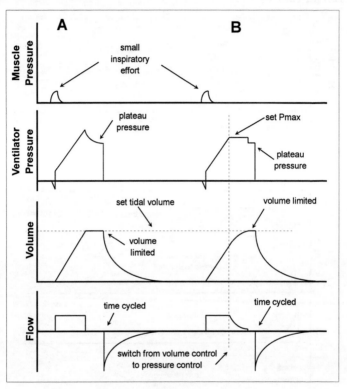

This figure compares VC-CMV with DC-CMV. (A) Volume controlled breath is patient triggered, volume and flow limited, and time cycled. (B) Dual controlled breath starting inspiration in volume control but switching to pressure control when airway pressure reaches the set P_{max}. Flow stops when the set tidal volume is met. An inspiratory hold ensues until the set inspiratory time is met and the breath is cycled off. Notice that the inspiratory flow time is increased while the inspiratory pause time is decreased to assure tidal volume delivery in the set inspiratory time. P_{max} results in a lower pressure at the airway opening but the same pressure in the lungs due to the same tidal volume as in the volume controlled breath. The Bear 1000 has an automatic dual control feature called "flow augmentation" that will allow a breath to start out in volume control but switches to pressure control if the patient makes an inspiratory effort that drops airway pressure below baseline. Both flow and volume may increase above the set values to meet the patient's demand and maintain the set baseline pressure.

Review and Consider

19. During VC-CMV, what happens to airway pressure when the patient makes an inspiratory effort throughout the inspiratory time?

20. During DC-CMV, how does the ventilator know the difference between an improvement in lung compliance and a greater inspiratory effort?

21. Explain the difference between the dual control between breaths and dual control within breaths.

22. What is the difference between DC-CMV between breaths and DC-CMV within breaths in terms of the parameters you have to set on the ventilator?

23. Explain the difference between dual control between breaths and dual control within breaths in terms of the set and actual pressure and volume.

24. For both types of dual control within breaths, what happens to inspiratory time when the control variable switches?

25. During Volume Assured Pressure Support or Pressure Augmentation, what happens if you set the pressure limit too high or low relative to the set tidal volume? What happens if you set the flow too high or low relative to the set tidal volume?

Intermittent Mandatory Ventilation (IMV)

VC-IMV (unassisted spontaneous breaths)

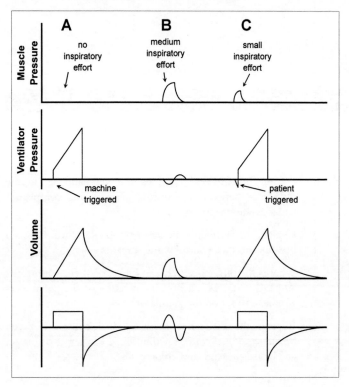

Mandatory breaths may be time triggered (A) or patient triggered (C). When patient triggering is allowed, this mode is often referred to as synchronized IMV or SIMV. Unassisted spontaneous breaths may occur between mandatory breaths (B). The small fluctuation in airway pressure during spontaneous breaths is due to the resistance of the expiratory limb of the patient circuit.

VC-IMV (assisted spontaneous breaths)

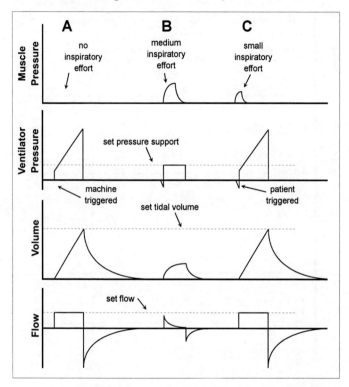

Mandatory breaths may be time triggered (A) or patient triggered (C). When patient triggering is allowed, this mode is often referred to as synchronized IMV or SIMV. Assisted spontaneous breaths may occur between mandatory breaths (B).

PC-IMV

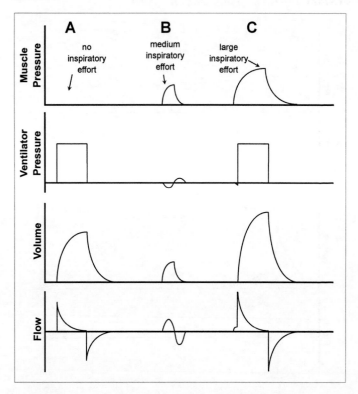

Mandatory breaths may be time triggered (A) or patient triggered (C). When patient triggering is allowed, this mode is often referred to as synchronized IMV or SIMV. Spontaneous breaths may occur between mandatory breaths (B). The example shown is unassisted, but assisted mandatory breaths are possible. The small fluctuation in airway pressure during spontaneous breaths are due to the resistance of the expiratory limb of the patient circuit.

DC-IMV

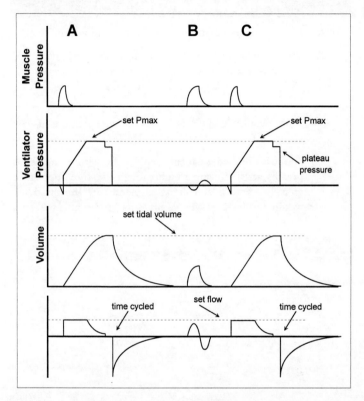

Mandatory breaths (A and C) may be any type of dual control as shown previously. Spontaneous breaths may occur between mandatory breaths (B). Spontaneous breaths may be unassisted as shown or assisted (as in Pressure Support). The small fluctuation in airway pressure during spontaneous breaths is due to the resistance of the expiratory limb of the patient circuit.

Review and Consider

26. How are spontaneous breaths assisted during IMV?

27. What would you expect the effect on tidal volume would be if a neonate was switched from machine triggered PC-IMV to patient triggered PC-IMV (that is, from IMV to SIMV)?

28. What would happen to mean airway pressure if you switched from VC-CMV to VC-IMV?

29. Suppose you had a patient on VC-IMV with spontaneous breaths assisted using a high enough Pressure Support to give the same tidal volume as mandatory breaths. How would the level of ventilatory support be affected by a decrease in the IMV rate?

Continuous Spontaneous Ventilation (CSV)

Continuous Positive Airway Pressure (CPAP)

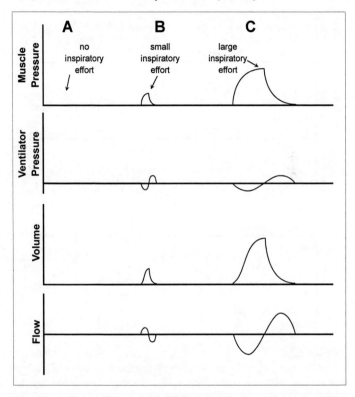

Continuous positive airway pressure allows the patient to breathe at a constant pressure above atmospheric pressure (A). Breaths are unassisted. In fact, any changes in airway pressure (B and C) occur because CPAP systems are never perfect pressure controllers. A drop in airway pressure during inspiration and a rise during expiration are indications that the patient is doing work on the CPAP circuit. A good pressure controller will keep the pressure fluctuations at a minimum regardless of the patient's inspiratory effort (see B compared to C).

Pressure Support

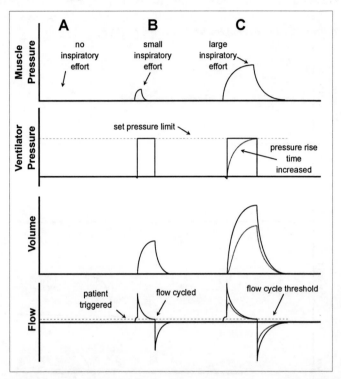

Pressure Support is a form of continuous spontaneous ventilation in which breaths are pressure or flow triggered, pressure limited, and flow cycled. Usually the flow cycle threshold is preset by the manufacturer as a percentage of peak flow or perhaps as an absolute flow setting. Some ventilators allow the operator to set the flow cycle threshold or even the pressure rise time to improve patient synchrony. Rise time (the time required to reach the pressure limit) affects the shape of the pressure waveform. A short rise time gives a more rectangular shape while a long rise time gives a more triangular shape (C). Increasing the rise time decreases the mean inspiratory pressure, which in turn decreases the peak flow and tidal volume. When the rise time is set too short, inspiration is prematurely terminated. When it is set too long, inspiratory flow is too low and inspiratory time prolonged.

Proportional Assist

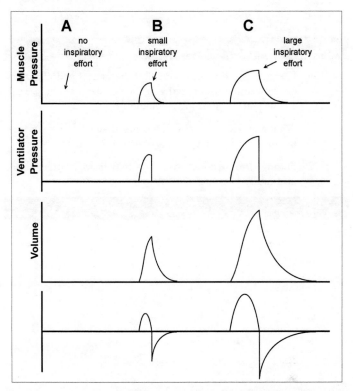

In this mode, the ventilator produces inspiratory pressure in proportion to the patient's effort. As the patient increases inspiratory effort, both flow, tidal volume, and inspiratory time all increase. For a given tidal volume and flow, the peak pressure depends on how much of the patient's elastance and resistance the operator has set the ventilator to bear.

Review and Consider

30. During CSV, how can you tell if the patient is doing work on the ventilator to breathe or the ventilator is doing work on the patient (assisting inspiration)?

31. What happens to tidal volume and flow when you change the pressure rise time during Pressure Support?

32. During Proportional Assist, what factors affect peak inspiratory pressure?

How to Detect problems

Assessing Overall Quality

Appropriate Scales

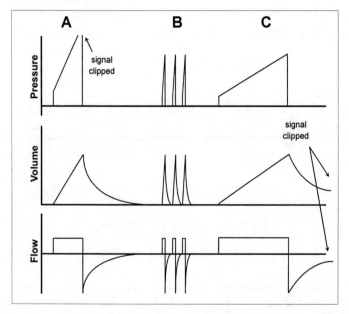

(A) The pressure scale is too small and the waveform is cut-off or "clipped". You cannot see the peak inspiratory pressure. (B) The sweep speed is too slow. This makes the time scale too long and you lose detail in the waveforms. (C) The sweep speed is too fast. The time scale is too short, the expiratory waveforms are clipped and you cannot see a whole breath. These problems are avoided with ventilator monitors that automatically adjust scales. You may run into these problems with stand alone monitors or if you are doing research using strip chart recorders.

Leak

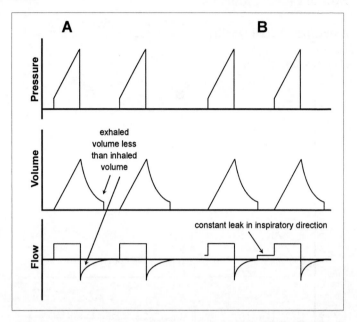

(A) Intermittent leak, as through a chest tube or around an uncuffed endotracheal tube. Volume leaks out mostly during inspiration when pressure is elevated and the airways are dilated. The volume waveform abruptly returns to zero because the integrator resets when the software thinks expiration has ended (when flow crosses zero). However, it is clear that the height of the inspiratory portion of the volume curve is bigger than the expiratory portion. Flow returns to zero but the area under the flow curve (which is proportional to volume) is smaller for expiration than inspiration. These are both signs that the exhaled volume is less than the inhaled volume. (B) Constant leak. Notice the same signs of leak as in (A) but the leak is present throughout the breath. This is indicated by the expiratory flow curve that remains above zero, indicating a constant positive (inspiratory direction) flow. Large leaks in the patient circuit or through a chest tube may do this. The CPAP level may be reduced by a large leak if the ventilator cannot compensate.

Assessing for Optimum Settings

Sensitivity

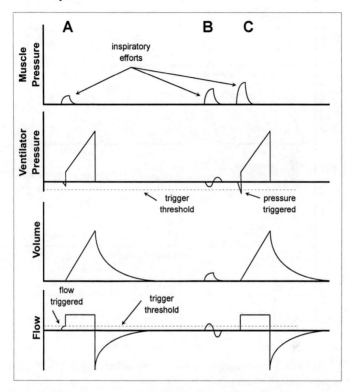

(A) Appropriately set sensitivity for flow triggering. A small patient effort results in an inspiratory flow signal that crosses the triggering threshold and starts inspiration. There is a small pressure drop because the exhalation manifold is open. (B) Inappropriately set sensitivity for pressure triggering. A fairly large inspiratory effort fails to drop airway pressure below the triggering threshold. The resulting volume and flow are very small because the exhalation manifold is closed. (C) The patient makes a larger effort and now the pressure drops below the triggering threshold to start inspiration. If the pressure drop is more than 2 cm H_2O, the setting is probably not sensitive enough.

Inspiratory Flow Too Low

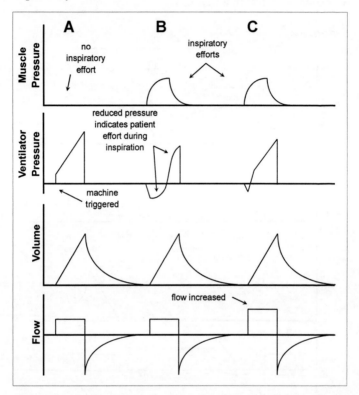

(A) Machine (time) triggered, volume controlled breath. (B) Patient triggered breath during which delivered flow was inadequate to unload the muscles fully. Area between pressure curve and time axis below baseline pressure is proportional to the work the patient does on the ventilator. (C) Inspiratory flow increased to unload the muscles. Switching to a pressure control or dual control mode would also eliminate this problem.

Notice that the work the patient does on the ventilator in (C) is just enough to trigger inspiration. However, the muscles still do work as indicated by the lower peak and mean inspiratory pressure. (Mean inspiratory pressure is proportional to the area between the pressure curve and the time axis.)

Review and Consider

33. How can you tell the difference between an intermittent and a continuous leak?

34. How could you tell by looking at the graphic waveforms whether a ventilator was pressure or flow triggered?

35. The graphic on the right was taken from an article in Respiratory Care. It shows pressure (top), flow (middle) and volume (bottom) during a *mandatory* breath. The author claims, "The slightly concave appearance of the pressure trace (arrow) indicates that flow toward the end of the breath does not meet the patient demand".

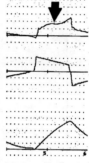

a. What mode of ventilation is this?

b. Do you agree with the author's claim? Explain your answer in terms of the ideas shown on the previous page.

Inspiratory Time Too Short

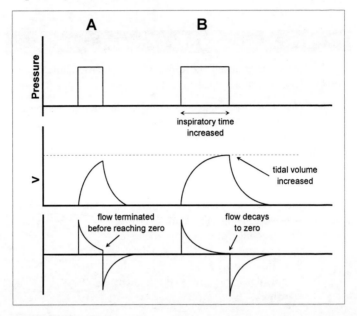

During pressure controlled ventilation, inspiratory time must last at least 5 time constants in order for the maximum (99.3 %) tidal volume to be delivered with the set pressure limit. (A) Inspiratory time is set too short to deliver the maximum possible tidal volume. This can be seen by observing that the inspiratory flow curve is cut off prematurely. (B) Inspiratory time has been extended, allowing flow to decay to zero and thereby increasing tidal volume.

Expiratory Time Too Short (autoPEEP)

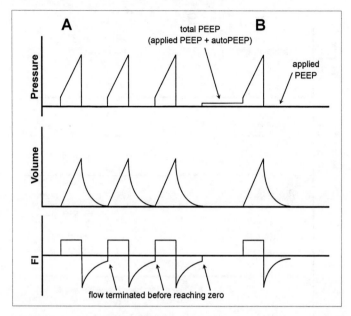

Expiratory time must be at least 5 time constants long to avoid gas trapping. (A) Expiratory time is too short, resulting in gas trapping and autoPEEP. This is indicated by the expiratory flow curve being abruptly cut off before it decays to zero. The cause may be that the frequency is too high or there is an elevated expiratory resistance, such as collapsed airways or endotracheal tube kinking. (B) After the third breath, the airway was occluded using the end-expiratory hold function of the ventilator. During the period of zero flow, pressures in the lung and ventilator circuit equilibrate. The static airway pressure then represents total PEEP.

$$total\ PEEP = applied\ PEEP + autoPEEP$$

$$autoPEEP = total\ PEEP - applied\ PEEP$$

Asynchrony (PC-IMV)

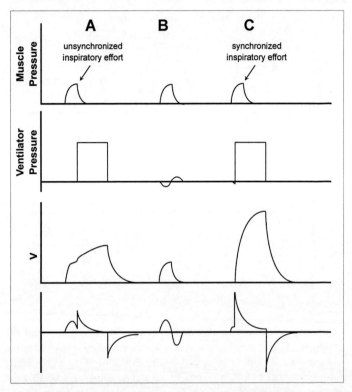

Asynchrony is common during pressure controlled ventilation of neonates. (A) The ventilator triggers a mandatory breath at the end of a spontaneous inspiration. As a result, the patient cannot exhale as expected and inspiratory time is prolonged. (B) An unassisted spontaneous breath. (C) A mandatory breath is time triggered coincidentally with a spontaneous effort. As a result, inspiratory flow and volume are larger and inspiratory time is shorter than the unsynchronized breath in A. Note that asynchrony in PC-IMV may lead to inconsistent tidal volumes and unstable gas exchange and blood gases.

Asynchrony (closed exhalation valve)

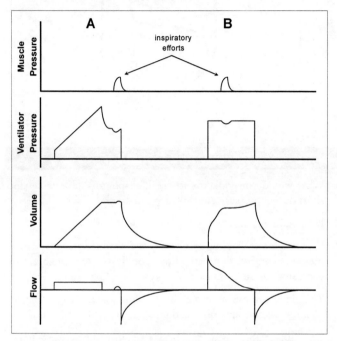

(A) Patient inspiratory effort late in *volume controlled* inspiration causes a pressure distortion during the inspiratory hold. (B) Patient inspiratory effort during *pressure controlled* inspiration distorts pressure waveform. In each case, the ventilator has closed the exhalation manifold so the patient can get no substantial volume or flow from these extra inspiratory efforts (only what is available from the gas compressed in the patient circuit). This type of asynchrony imposes unnecessary work on the patient. It can be eliminated by switching to a mode that allows the patient to breathe freely after a mandatory inspiration has been triggered. The Flow Augment feature on the Bear 1000 (volume control) and the BiLevel mode on the Puritan Bennett 840 (pressure control) are examples of ventilators that have addressed this problem. Switching to a dual control mode (such as Adaptive Support Ventilation on the Hamilton Galileo) may be an even better solution because it requires less adjustment by the operator.

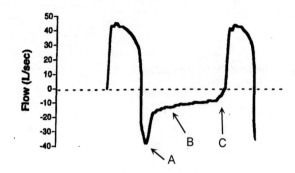

Review and Consider

36. What would you look for to see if inspiratory time is set too short during pressure controlled ventilation?

37. How can you tell if expiratory time is set too short?

38. If a patient makes an inspiratory effort during a mandatory pressure controlled breath, how could you tell whether the ventilator has an "active exhalation valve"?

39. The graphic above shows an actual flow tracing from a patient with obstructive lung disease during mechanical ventilation.

    a. Initially there is a high peak expiratory flow (A). What is the most probable cause of this?

    b. Flow throughout most of expiration is slow and linear rather than exponential (B). What does this suggest?

    c. If you saw oscillations in the flow waveform throughout expiration, what might that suggest?

    d. What does the abrupt transition from expiratory to inspiratory flow (C) suggest?

Loop Displays

Loop displays plot one control variable against another as compared to waveform displays that plot individual control variables against time. This allows a rapid assessment of the patient's respiratory system compliance and resistance. Recall that compliance is the change in volume for a given change in pressure. Graphically, that is equivalent to the slope of a curve with pressure on the horizontal axis and volume on the vertical axis. Thus, plotting the pressure-volume curves for inspiration and expiration yield information about compliance. Resistance is assessed from a plot of volume versus flow. As with the waveform displays, we will discuss idealized loops first and then show how real loops look. Then we will review briefly the ways loops may be interpreted.

Pressure-Volume Loop

Pressure-volume loops are commonly used both in clinical situations and for research purposes.

Key Idea

> There are two distinct types of pressure-volume loop and it is very important not to confuse them. They are the *static pressure-volume loop* and the *dynamic pressure-volume loop*. The static loop has been used by physiologists to describe lung characteristics for decades. It is produced by injecting an isolated set of lungs or the intact respiratory system with known amounts of gas and recording the associated pressures. In practice, a large, calibrated "super syringe" is used to deliver incremental volumes of 50 to 100 mL from functional residual volume up to total lung capacity (TLC). Static airway pressure is measured following a 1 to 2 second pause after each volume increment. Stepwise inflation is continued up to a predetermined maximum pressure (usually about 35-40 cm H_2O, which normally corresponds to TLC). The same measurements are made during stepwise deflation. Corrections for temperature, humidity, compressible volume and pulmonary gas exchange are required for accurate volume measurement.

The purpose of the pauses between volume increments is to remove any effects of resistance on the pressure measurements. That way, the pressure volume curve can be used to assess respiratory system compliance. This is a cumbersome clinical procedure because it requires that the patient be paralyzed, disconnected from the ventilator and stable enough to last through the whole process. Unfortunately, the patients you most want the data from are often so sick they cannot tolerate the procedure. An alternative technique is to inflate the lungs steadily with a very low constant flow (1-2 L/min). With the slow flow, resistance effects are negligible. This not only speeds up the procedure somewhat but also makes it possible for the ventilator to do it automatically. To date, only one ventilator has this capability (Hamilton Galileo).

You will note that the static pressure-volume curve of the lungs is different for inflation compared to deflation, which gives the "loop" appearance. The separation of the two curves is called hysteresis. Specifically, for each volume increment, there is less elastic recoil pressure during deflation than inflation and the volume returned during deflation is less than the inflation volume. All elastic materials show this type of behavior when stretched and released, but lung hysteresis is thought to be mainly due to oxygen being absorbed from the lung at a greater rate than carbon dioxide is excreted. Expansion of collapsed alveoli may also play a part.

The dynamic pressure-volume curve is what you see on ventilator monitors during normal mechanical ventilation. It is simply a plot of airway pressure on the horizontal axis versus volume on the vertical axis at normal inspiratory and expiratory flows. Consequently, the curves include effects from both compliance and resistance and they must be interpreted differently from static curves.

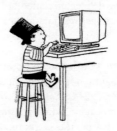

"A computer lets you make more mistakes
faster than any invention, with the possible
exceptions of handguns and tequila."
Mitch Rathliffe

Static Pressure-Volume Loop (compliance curves)

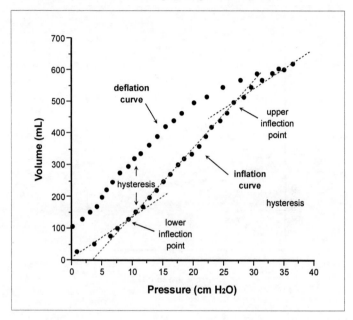

This graph shows the static pressure-volume curve of a patient with ARDS. The dotted lines represent areas of approximately linear compliance. The slope of a line is the compliance:

$$slope = \Delta\ volume / \Delta\ pressure = compliance$$

Idea

Maximum compliance is found between the two inflection points. This is where tidal ventilation should occur to minimize lung damage. An inflection point is a transition from one linear compliance to another. Compliance is less below the lower inflection point due to alveolar collapse. Compliance above the upper inflection point is also less due to alveolar over-distention. There is no universally accepted technique for determining the inflection points and it is often done visually. Also, inflection points are not always evident on any particular patient.

Static Pressure-Volume Curve (optimum ventilator settings)

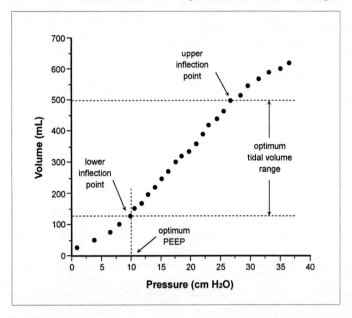

There are some clinical data to suggest that PEEP should be set above the lower inflection point to maximize oxygenation and minimize lung injury due to repeated collapse and expansion of lung tissue during the breathing cycle. Keep in mind that while such a PEEP level may be "optimum" in terms of compliance and PaO_2, it may not be the best for cardiac output and hence oxygen delivery to the tissues.

It is advisable to keep tidal volume below the upper inflection point to minimize the risk of lung damage due to over-distention.

Dynamic Pressure-Volume Loop (idealized; volume control)

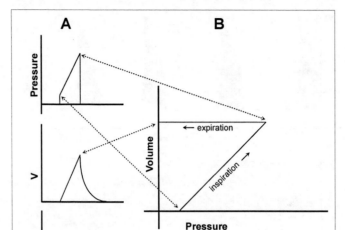

Idealized waveforms (A) for volume controlled ventilation with corresponding idealized pressure-volume loop (B). Note that the loop is drawn counterclockwise, with inspiration going to the right and up and expiration to the left and down. The dotted arrows show the correspondence between the waveform display and the loop display for the initial pressure rise, peak pressure, and tidal volume. After the initial pressure rise (when volume is zero) volume and pressure rise together to give a slanted line on the pressure-volume curve.

Key Idea

> Recall that the initial pressure rise is due mainly to the product of resistance and initial flow. Therefore, the lower inflection point on the *dynamic* pressure-volume curve does not correspond to an optimum PEEP level.

On expiration, the airway pressure drops immediately to zero. The shape of the expiratory portion of the pressure-volume loop is dominated by the fact that pressure is zero, which hides any effect of volume change. This results in a horizontal line.

Dynamic Pressure-Volume Loop (real; volume control)

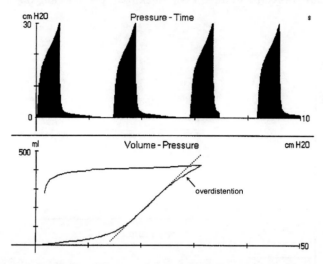

The figure above shows the actual pressure-time waveforms and pressure-volume loop from a ventilator monitor during volume controlled ventilation. Note that the airway pressure rises more gradually in these pressure-time waveforms than on an idealized waveform. This is due to patient circuit compliance and delays in the flow control valve. As a result, the lower inflection point on the pressure-volume curve is raised off the horizontal axis and is more rounded. Again, the lower inflection point is not indicative of airway collapse/recruitment or of optimal PEEP. It has little practical use on a dynamic pressure-volume loop.

Note also that airway pressure does not return to baseline immediately on the pressure time waveform. This is due to resistance through the expiratory portion of the patient circuit. As a result, there is a curvature in the expiratory portion of the pressure-volume loop.

There is a visible upper inflection point that might indicate over-distention and a need to reduce the tidal volume. (The dotted line was drawn by hand to help visualize the inflection points). Over-distention is also suggested on the pressure-time waveform by the concave upward shape of the inspiratory pressure after the initial pressure rise.

Dynamic Pressure-Volume Curve (idealized; pressure control)

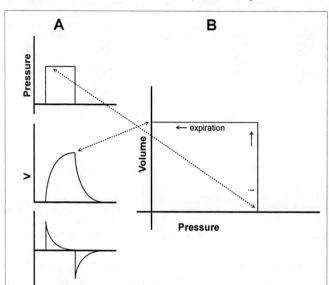

Idealized waveforms (A) for pressure controlled ventilation with corresponding idealized pressure-volume loop (B). Note that the loop is drawn counterclockwise. The dotted arrows show the correspondence between the waveform display and the loop display for the peak pressure and tidal volume. The shape of the inspiratory pressure-volume loop is dominated by the fact that pressure rises immediately to the pressure limit before volume starts to increase. The result is a vertical line, which eliminates any possibility of seeing either a lower or upper inflection point.

On expiration, the airway pressure drops immediately to zero. The shape of the expiratory portion of the pressure-volume loop is dominated by the fact that pressure is zero, which hides any effect of volume change. This results in a horizontal line.

Dynamic Pressure-Volume Curve (real; pressure control)

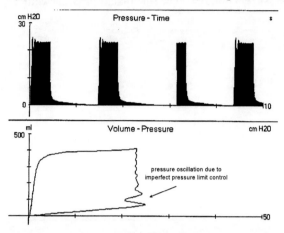

Actual pressure-time waveforms and pressure-volume loop from a ventilator monitor during pressure controlled ventilation. Note that the airway pressure rises more gradually in these pressure-time waveforms than on an idealized waveform. This is due to patient circuit compliance and delays in the flow control valve. As a result, the lower inflection point on the pressure-volume curve is raised off the horizontal axis and is more rounded. There is also an oscillation due to the imperfect pressure control of a real ventilator. Again, the lower inflection point is not indicative of airway collapse/recruitment or of optimal PEEP. It has little practical use on a dynamic pressure-volume loop.

Note also that airway pressure does not return to baseline immediately on the pressure time waveform. This is due to resistance through the expiratory portion of the patient circuit, producing a curvature in the expiratory portion of the pressure-volume loop.

Key Idea

Pressure waveforms during pressure control are highly variable. To the extent that the waveform is rectangular (rather than triangular or exponential) the inspiratory portion of the pressure-volume curve will tend to be straight and vertical. As a result, there may be little or no indication of over-distention even if a significant amount is really present.

Dynamic Pressure-Volume Curve (C_{20}/C_{dyn} index)

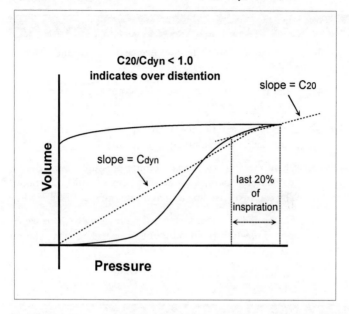

Some ventilator monitors quantitate over-distention by calculating the C_{20}/C_{dyn} index. C_{dyn} is **dynamic compliance**, defined as the slope of the pressure-volume curve drawn between two points of zero flow (which occur the start and end of inspiration). The C_{20} is compliance of the last 20% of inspiration. If the C_{20} is less than C_{dyn} (as in the figure above, indicated by the C_{20} line being more horizontal than the C_{dyn} line), their ratio will be less than 1.0, indicating over-distention. A ratio of greater than 1.0 indicates that the pressure-volume curve cannot be used to assess over-distention. This will happen during pressure controlled ventilation where the ventilator attempts to maintain a constant inspiratory pressure (at least near end inspiration) and hence the pressure-volume loop at end inspiration is nearly vertical.

Review and Consider

40. How do you calculate compliance from a static volume-pressure curve?

41. What is an inflection point? How could you identify one on a volume-pressure curve?

42. Explain the significance of the upper and lower inflection points on a *static* volume-pressure curve.

43. When viewing a *dynamic* volume-pressure curve during ventilation you may often see a lower inflection point. Why can't you use this to determine optimal PEEP?

44. What is the problem associated with trying to visualize an upper inflection point on a volume-pressure curve during pressure controlled ventilation?

45. Explain the significance and interpretation of the C_{20}/C_{dyn} index.

Flow-Volume Loop

Flow-volume loops have traditionally been used in the pulmonary function lab to diagnose lung disease. Flow-volume loops generated during mechanical ventilation are different in three major respects from those obtained in the pulmonary function lab:

1. Flow-volume loops obtained during mechanical ventilation are normally passive, compared to the forced vital capacity maneuver required of patients in the lab.

2. The shape of the inspiratory portion of the loop during mechanical ventilation is determined by the flow waveform generated by the ventilator.

3. The expiratory portion of the loop does reflect changes in airway resistance but does not necessarily indicate maximal flow limitation as in pulmonary function studies.

Unfortunately, there is no consensus on how the axes should be oriented. Sometimes flow is shown on the vertical scale and sometimes on the horizontal scale. Sometimes inspiration is shown as a positive (upward) flow and sometimes it is downward. *This book will show flow on the vertical scale with inspiration in the positive, upward direction.*

Flow-volume loops can be used to detect autoPEEP and leaks like waveforms can, but they are most useful in the evaluation of bronchodilator response. As you will see below, examination of the expiratory portion of the flow-volume loop clearly shows a change in the shape of the curve as resistance changes. Another practical use of flow-volume waveforms is to access asynchrony during pressure controlled ventilation of neonates. If the infant breathes spontaneously, and out of phase with mandatory breaths, tidal volume delivery will be highly variable. This problem can be minimized by proper setting of the sensitivity. If SIMV is not available, it is sometimes possible to set the IMV frequency such that the patient's rate is "entrained" (the patient is stimulated to breathe at the same rate or some even multiple of the ventilator rate, thus increasing synchrony). Synchrony between the patient and ventilator and the resultant decrease in tidal volume variability is easily seen with flow-volume loops that overlap for several breaths. Low tidal volume variability is desirable not only to stabilize gas exchange but also to minimize the risk of intracranial bleeds.

Volume Control (idealized)

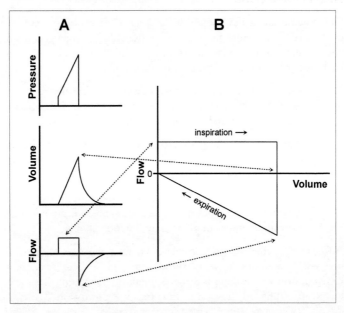

Idealized waveforms (A) for volume controlled ventilation with corresponding idealized flow-volume loop (B). Note that the loop is drawn clockwise, with inspiration going to the right and down and expiration to the left and up. The dotted arrows show the correspondence between the waveform display and the loop display for the initial flow rise and tidal volume. The shape of the inspiratory portion of the flow-volume loop is dominated by the constant flow, which hides the change in volume and results in a horizontal line.

During expiration, both volume and flow decrease exponentially with the same time constant (see the discussion about time constants in Chapter 4). When one exponential function is plotted against another and there is a single time constant for the system, the result is a straight line. This can be proven mathematically but you can understand it intuitively by recognizing that if volume and flow are changing at the same rate (having the same time constant) then the ratio of flow to volume (the slope of the expiratory portion of the flow-volume curve) must remain constant. A curve with a constant slope is a straight line.

Volume Control (real; normal vs. COPD)

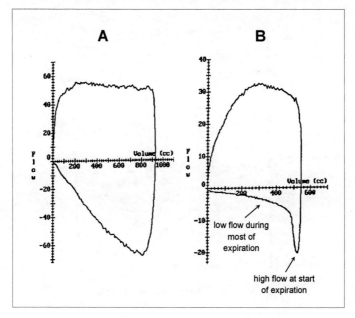

Actual flow-volume loop from a ventilator monitor during volume controlled ventilation of a normal patient (A) and one with chronic obstructive lung disease, COPD (B).

Patients with normal lungs have relatively straight expiratory curves while those with marked airway collapse (like COPD patients) may show a biphasic curve. If the expiratory portion of the curve is not a straight line, it indicates that the respiratory system really does not behave as if it has only a single time constant. In patients with lung disease, lung units will be affected to different degrees and each will have its own time constant.

The high flow at the start of expiration in B is due to the gas compressed in the patient circuit. The relatively low flow for the rest of expiration comes from the lungs and may represent flow limitation due to collapsed airways.

Volume Control (real; pre-post bronchodilator)

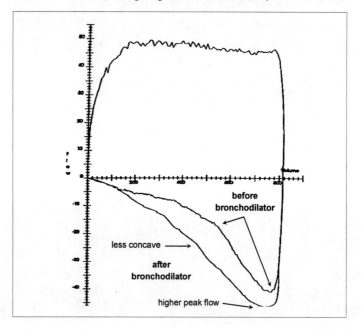

Actual flow-volume loop from a ventilator monitor during volume controlled ventilation of an asthmatic patient. Note the obvious response to bronchodilator therapy as indicated by the higher peak expiratory flow and the decrease in the concavity of the expiratory flow-volume curve.

Pressure Control (idealized)

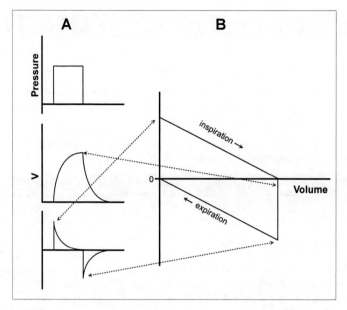

Idealized waveforms (A) for pressure controlled ventilation with corresponding idealized flow-volume loop (B). Note that the loop is drawn clockwise, with inspiration going to the right and down and expiration to the left and up. The dotted arrows show the correspondence between the waveform display and the loop display for the initial flow rise and tidal volume. The shape of the inspiratory portion of the flow-volume loop is the mirror image of the expiratory portion just as the volume-time and flow-time curves are mirror images when comparing inspiration with expiration.

During inspiration and expiration, both volume and flow change exponentially with the same time constant (see the discussion about time constants in Chapter 4). When one exponential function is plotted against another and there is a single time constant for the system, the result is a straight line. This can be proven mathematically but you can understand it intuitively by recognizing that if volume and flow are changing at the same rate (ie, the same time constant) then the ratio of flow to volume (the slope of the expiratory portion of the flow-volume curve) must remain constant. A curve with a constant slope is a straight line.

46. On a flow-volume loop, what determines the shape of the inspiratory portion of the loop?

47. How does the expiratory portion of a flow-volume loop differ between a normal patient and one with chronic obstructive lung disease?

48. Using flow-volume loops, how could you determine if a bronchodilator treatment was effective?

Calculated Parameters

Most of the ventilators that provide graphic displays also show various calculated parameters. Unfortunately, ventilator operator's manuals do not always define these terms or explain the equations used. The following parameters are the most common.

Mean Airway Pressure

Mean airway pressure is defined as the average pressure at the airway opening over a given time interval. It is defined graphically as the area under the pressure time curve for one breath cycle divided by the total cycle time. If all breaths are identical, then the average pressure for one breath is the average over any period. However, because mandatory breaths may be mixed with spontaneous breaths and because the pressure waveforms for each of these may change on a breath-by-breath basis, mean airway pressure is usually calculated as a moving average over several breath cycles. The ventilator measures airway pressure every few milliseconds for a few breath cycles. Then it sums the measurements and divides by the number of measurements to get the average. The average is "moving" because as the measurements for the next breaths come in, they replace those of the first breaths in the average. For example, the Hamilton Galileo calculates mean airway pressure as the moving average of 8 breath cycles. In contrast, the Puritan Bennett 840 displays mean airway pressure for each breath.

Figure 5-8 shows two ways to calculate mean airway pressure. The graphical method is based on the mean value theorem from calculus.[5] This theorem says that the mean value of a periodic waveform is the constant value that will give the same area as the waveform over the same period. The area under the waveform on the left in Figure 5-8 can be represented by the number of boxes between the pressure curve and the time axis. Notice that the constant (mean) pressure on the right has the same area.

The numerical method is used by ventilators and is just the arithmetic average of a large number of pressure measurements. The shorter the sampling period, the larger the number of pressure measurements the more closely the waveform is followed and the more accurate the estimate of mean airway pressure. This method may be extended over several breaths to give a moving average that does not change as quickly as a breath-by-breath display.

Mean airway pressure can also be estimated by hand based only on peak inspiratory pressure (PIP), positive end expiratory pressure (PEEP) and the duty cycle:

$$\overline{P}_{AW} = k(PIP - PEEP)(T_I / TCT) + PEEP$$

where k is the waveform constant, T_I = inspiratory time and TCT is total cycle time (respiratory period). The waveform constant can take on any value from 1.0 for a rectangular waveform (pressure control ventilation) to 0.5 for a triangular waveform (volume control ventilation). The shorter the pressure rise time, the larger k will be. This equation was developed years ago, before ventilators routinely displayed mean airway pressure. In practice, the value of k was determined experimentally by graphically calculating mean airway pressure for a given type of ventilator mode and then using the value for subsequent estimation of mean airway pressure based only on the ventilator settings. The main value of the equation today is to show what factors are important in determining mean airway pressure.

---

[5] Crit Care Med 1982;10(6):378-383.

Figure 5-8. Two methods of calculating mean airway pressure.

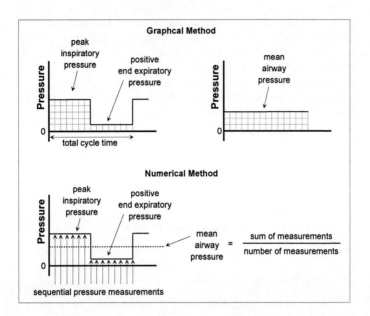

Leak

The leak volume is the difference between the inspired tidal volume and the expired volume. It may be a moving average calculated over several breaths. This value is particularly important in patients with uncuffed endotracheal tubes or with broncho-pleural-cutaneous fistulas.

Calculating Respiratory System Mechanics: Static vs. Dynamic

There are two methods used to calculate compliance and resistance at the bedside; a static method and a dynamic method. Both of these methods rely on pressure measurements taken at the airway opening. As we have discussed many times, airway pressure has two components, one due to compliance and volume; the other due to resistance and flow. The technical problem in calculating mechanics is to separate these two components without having to make pressure measurements within the lung in order to obtain transairway pressure for resistance and transthoracic pressure for compliance. The solution is to make the measurements in such a way that the pressure measured at the airway opening reflects only the component of interest. The "trick" is to realize that we are measuring a change in pressure not only between two points in space (at the airway opening and in the lung), but also between two points in time.

The static method accomplishes this by taking measurements at the start of inspiration (when flow and volume are zero) and at the end of an inspiratory hold maneuver (when flow is zero and volume is the tidal volume). Because flow is zero at both times, airway pressure is the same as the pressure in the lung. The pressure change between those times is due only to the volume change. Compliance can then be calculated as the volume change (tidal volume) divided by the airway pressure change (plateau pressure minus PEEP).

In a similar fashion, if we take measurements at two times when flow is different but volume is the same, we can calculate resistance. These two times are at the end of inspiratory flow time and at the end of inspiratory hold time. Thus, resistance is simply the pressure change (peak inspiratory pressure minus plateau pressure) divided by the change in flow. The change in flow is the flow at the end of the inspiratory flow time minus the flow at end expiratory time (zero) which simplifies to just the end inspiratory flow.

The dynamic method of calculating respiratory system mechanics was designed for situations when an inspiratory hold is not practical. The basic idea is still the same; compliance is assessed by making measurements of pressure between two points in time when flow is zero (start and end inspiration) and resistance is assessed between two points in time when volumes are equal. However, because we do not have the luxury of a few milliseconds of inspiratory hold to read the pressure values from the ventilator's gauge, we need to analyze pressure, volume, and flow waveforms. Pressure measurements for compliance are read off the graph at times when the flow waveform crosses zero. Pressure measurements for resistance are read off the graph at times when the volumes are equal, usually mid inspiration and mid expiration.

While the dynamic method described above has been used extensively for research, it is not very practical for routing bedside calculations. For that reason, ventilator manufacturers have made use of the microprocessor's capability of making rapid measurements and calculations to simplify things. Because the ventilator is already making continuous pressure, volume and flow measurements for control and alarm purposes, they simply use that data for the additional purpose of calculating resistance and compliance. This is done by fitting the equation of motion to the data using linear regression as described in the next section. The advantage of this, besides being automated, is that both inspiratory and expiratory parameters can be calculated on a breath-by-breath basis without disturbing the patient's breathing pattern.

Compliance

Compliance is the constant of proportionality between volume and pressure for the respiratory system. There are two methods used to calculate compliance; a static method and a dynamic method. The static method (Figure 5-9) requires either an automatic or a manually created inspiratory hold during volume controlled ventilation.

Figure 5-9. Static compliance measurement.

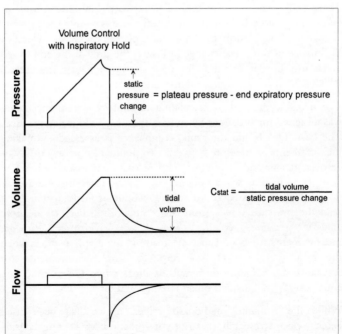

Compliance is estimated as the tidal volume divided by the difference between plateau pressure and end expiratory pressure. End expiratory pressure is either PEEP or, if there is gas trapping, total PEEP. If the tidal volume is not measured at the airway opening, and includes the volume compressed in the patient circuit, the compliance of the patient circuit must be subtracted from the total static compliance calculated as shown in Figure 5-9. Recall that the patient circuit and the respiratory system compliance are connected in parallel and parallel compliances are additive.

The dynamic method of estimating compliance makes use of a statistical procedure called least squares regression. The idea is illustrated in Figure 5-10 for a very simple data set of four pairs of volume-pressure measurements. A straight line is "fit" to the data by a mathematical procedure that minimizes the sum of the vertical distances from the data points to the line. The equation of the line in this case is

$$pressure = \frac{volume}{compliance}$$

The slope of the line is defined as compliance (mL/cmH$_2$O):

$$slope = compliance = \frac{\Delta volume}{\Delta pressure}$$

Figure 5-10. The least squares regression method for calculating compliance. The linear regression line is fit to the data by a mathematical procedure that minimizes the sum of the squared vertical distances between the data points and the line.

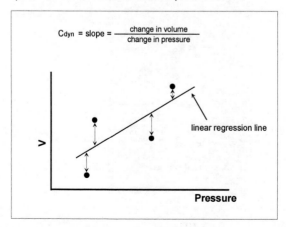

In practice, many sets of simultaneous pressure, volume, and flow measurements are made during the breath. Then, the regression technique is used to derive the constants (compliance and resistance) in the equation of motion:

$$pressure = \frac{volume}{compliance} + resistance \times flow$$

Compliance obtained in this way is called dynamic compliance because it is calculated during motion of the respiratory system. However, it is an estimate of the static compliance defined earlier. For this reason, there is often confusion because there is no standardization in terminology; sometimes it is called C_{stat} and sometimes C_{dyn}. If the respiratory system were really just a single flow conducting tube connected to an elastic compartment, the two compliances would be equivalent. However, in injured or diseased lungs there are many areas with different time constants. In that case, dynamic compliance becomes frequency dependent, decreasing as respiratory frequency increases.

Dynamic Characteristic

The dynamic characteristic is a crude index of respiratory system mechanics that can be calculated by hand without an inspiratory hold maneuver. That is about the only advantage of this parameter. It reflects both resistance and compliance, so it is difficult to interpret the index in a clinical situation. Figure 5-11 shows how dynamic characteristic is calculated. Note that many textbooks incorrectly call this parameter "dynamic compliance", perhaps because it is a ratio of volume to pressure.

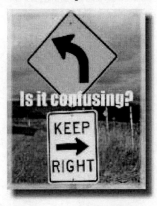

Figure 5-11. Calculation of the dynamic characteristic.

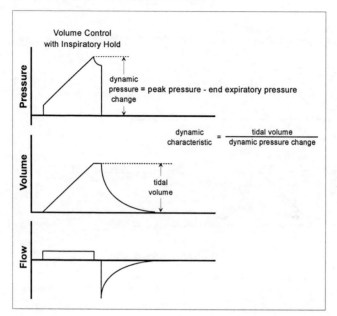

Resistance

Resistance is the constant of proportionality between pressure and flow for the respiratory system. There are two methods used to calculate resistance; a static method and a dynamic method. The static method (Figure 5-12) requires either an automatic or a manually created inspiratory hold during volume controlled ventilation. Resistance is then the difference between peak inspiratory pressure and plateau (static) pressure.

Figure 5-12. Static method of calculating resistance.

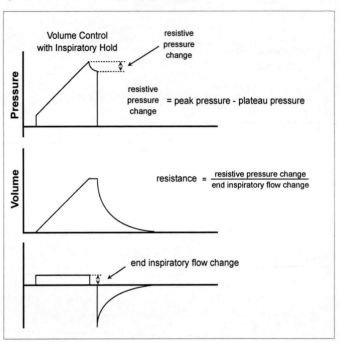

If the inspiratory flow is not measured at the airway opening, and includes the gas compressed in the patient circuit, the compliance of the patient circuit must be accounted for as follows:

$$R = \frac{\left(1 + \dfrac{C_{PC}}{C_{stat}}\right)\left(PIP - P_{stat}\right)}{\dot{V}}$$

where R = respiratory system (and endotracheal tube) resistance in $cmH_2O/L/s$, C_{PC} = patient circuit compliance, C_{stat} = static respiratory system compliance, PIP = peak inspiratory pressure, P_{stat} = static or plateau pressure during the inspiratory hold, $\dot{V}$ = end inspiratory flow.

The dynamic method of estimating compliance makes use of a statistical procedure called least squares regression. The equation of motion is "fit" to a set of data comprised of many pressure, volume, and flow measurements made during a breath. See the discussion for dynamic compliance above. This method makes it possible to separate out inspiratory resistance from expiratory resistance.

Review and Consider

49. In Figure 5-7 B, how can you verify the mean inspiratory pressure graphically (using analytic geometry rather than calculus)?

50. What are the three factors that affect mean airway pressure? Is it possible to change the frequency and not change the mean airway pressure?

51. How do ventilators usually calculate mean airway pressure?

52. Give the equations you would use to calculate resistance and compliance by hand at the bedside. How is this different from the way a ventilator would calculate the values if an inspiratory hold was not used?

Time Constant

The time constant was described in detail at the beginning of Chapter 4. It is defined as the time necessary for an exponential function to attain 63% of its steady state value. For example, passive exhalation is described by an exponential function. Therefore, when expiratory time reaches one time constant, 63% of the tidal volume will have been exhaled and expiratory flow will have decreased 63% from its peak value.

The time constant is calculated as the product of resistance and compliance:

$$\tau = RC$$

where the Greek letter tau, τ, is the time constant in seconds, R is resistance in cm $H_2O/L/s$ and C is compliance in L/cmH_2O.

Pressure-Time Product

The pressure-time product was originally defined as the integral of the pressure developed by the respiratory muscles (estimated using esophageal pressure) integrated over the duration of contraction. As such, it was intended as an index of respiratory work or the oxygen cost of breathing. There are many variations on this theme.

One ventilator, the Hamilton Galileo, displays a pressure time product they define as the integral of airway pressure from the time that pressure drops below baseline (during the triggering effort) until pressure crosses baseline again as flow is delivered from the ventilator:

$$PTP = \int_{0}^{T_{baseline}} P_{AW} \, dt$$

where PTP is the pressure time product in units of cmH_2O-seconds, $T_{baseline}$ is time that the airway pressure crosses the baseline pressure (PEEP or CPAP), P_{AW} is transrespiratory pressure and t is time. Graphically, this integral represents the area between the pressure curve and the time axis (see Figure 5-13). The pressure-time product calculated this way is an index of the work imposed on the patient to trigger the ventilator plus the work imposed by any delay the ventilator creates in delivering the flow demanded by the patient. A common example of when one might see a high PTP is when the patient's condition and the selection of mode and/or control settings are incompatible. For example, VC-CMV breath with low peak flow for a patient with strong respiratory drive and high peak flow demand. This patient might want 120 L/min but the clinician sets 60 L/min. The PTP will be large because the airway pressure will stay below baseline during inspiration until the patient's flow demand falls below 60 L/min. To a lesser extent, setting an inspiratory pressure limit too low during PC-CMV for the same patient might result in a large PTP. Dual control modes that auto regulate inspiratory flow to meet patient's demand will tend to result in a lower PTP than modes where the clinician must manually adjust the control settings to match the patient's ever changing flow demand.

Occlusion Pressure ($P_{0.1}$)

Airway occlusion pressure is defined as the value of airway pressure 0.1 seconds after initiation of an inspiratory effort against an occluded airway. It is a measure of the patient's central ventilatory drive. This index is relatively insensitive to changes in respiratory system mechanics and does not require scaling to patient size. Normal $P_{0.1}$ is about 1-2 cmH_2O during mechanical ventilation. Values above this indicate an increased ventilatory drive (the response of the respiratory centers to compromised pulmonary function) which may lead to exhaustion. Some data suggest that patients with $P_{0.1}$ values of 4-6 cmH_2O should not be weaned from the ventilator. The Drager Evita 4 calculates $P_{0.1}$ as shown in Figure 5-13.

Figure 5-13. Calculation of $P_{0.1}$ on the Drager Evita 4 ventilator. PTP = pressure-time product.

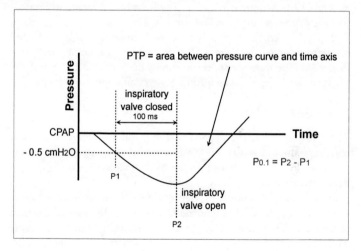

Rapid Shallow Breathing Index

This is an index used to predict which patients will be successfully weaned. It is calculated from measurements of spontaneous breathing frequency and tidal volume while the patient breathes unassisted (on a t-piece or on CPAP):

$$RSB\ Index = \frac{frequency}{tidal\ volume}$$

A value of ≤ 105 breaths/min/L predicts weaning success in adults. In children, the threshold value is < 11 breaths/min/mL/kg where tidal volume is expressed in mL/kg body weight.[6]

Inspiratory Force

Inspiratory force (sometimes called negative inspiratory force or NIF) is a measure of the maximum inspiratory effort against an occluded airway after a preceding expiration. It is an index used to predict which patients will be successfully weaned. Patients with an inspiratory force of more than -30 cmH$_2$O are likely to succeed while those with inspiratory force of 0 to -20 may not. The term "negative inspiratory force" can be confusing. A patient can have an inspiratory force of -30 cmH$_2$O or a negative inspiratory force of 30 cmH$_2$O but to say that a patient has a negative inspiratory force of -30 cmH$_2$O is a double negative. Furthermore, a larger inspiratory force is expressed by a smaller number. For example, an inspiratory force of -35 cmH$_2$O reflects a larger inspiratory effort than and inspiratory force of -30 cmH$_2$O, even though -35 is numerically less than -30. The number shows the magnitude of the force and the negative sign shows it is an inspiratory (versus expiratory) force.

AutoPEEP

The term autoPEEP is defined as the positive difference between end expiratory alveolar pressure and the end expiratory airway pressure (PEEP or CPAP) selected by the clinician. Total PEEP is thus intentionally applied PEEP or CPAP plus autoPEEP. AutoPEEP is the residual expiratory flow-driven pressure (pressure = resistance X flow) that remains just prior to the start of the next inspiration. There are several ways to measure autoPEEP. One method, used on the Drager Evita 4, is illustrated in Figure 5-14. The patient circuit compliance may affect the accuracy of the measurement (see the section on Effects of the Patient Circuit in Chapter 5).

---

[6] N Eng J Med 1991;324:1445-1450, Pediatr Pulmonol 1997;24:344-352

Figure 5-14. AutoPEEP and the volume of trapped gas measured during an expiratory hold maneuver. The airway is occluded at the point where the next breath would normally be triggered. During the brief occlusion period, the lung pressure equilibrates with the patient circuit to give a total PEEP reading. When the occlusion is released, the volume exhaled is the trapped gas.

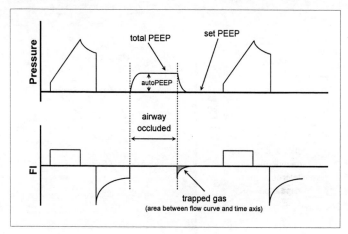

Work of Breathing

The general definition of work is the integral of pressure with respect to volume:

$$W = 0.098 \int P \, dv$$

where W is work in joules, 0.098 is the factor used to convert cmH_2O-L to joules, P is pressure and v is volume. It is conceptualized graphically as the area between the pressure curve and the volume axis on a volume pressure curve (Figure 5-15). Work is sometimes expressed as joules per liter of tidal volume.

There are two general kinds of work related to mechanical ventilation. One kind is the work performed by the ventilator on the patient, which is reflected by a positive change in airway pressure above baseline during inspiration. The other kind is the work the patient does on the ventilator (called the imposed work) to trigger inspiration.

Mechanical Ventilation

Figure 5-15. Work of breathing during mechanical ventilation. The patient does work on the ventilator as he inspires a small volume from the patient circuit and drops the airway pressure enough to trigger inspiration. The ventilator does work on the patient as airway pressure rises above baseline.

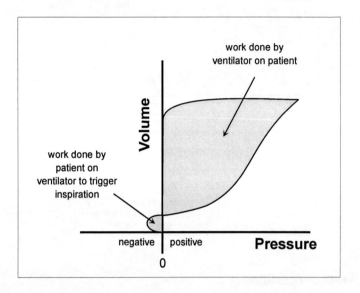

Review and Consider

53. What is the equation for calculating the time constant? What are its units of measurement?

54. Explain the difference between the pressure-time product and occlusion pressure ($P_{0.1}$).

55. The rapid shallow breathing index was designed for spontaneously breathing patients. Pressure Support is a form of continuous spontaneous ventilation. Is it appropriate to calculate the index during Pressure Support?

56. Is an inspiratory force of –35 cmH$_2$O more than or less than the value that is assumed to predict weaning success?

57. Explain the difference between applied PEEP, autoPEEP and total PEEP.

58. If you were looking at a pressure-volume loop, how would you visually assess the work of breathing imposed on the patient to trigger the ventilator?

Early model iron lung

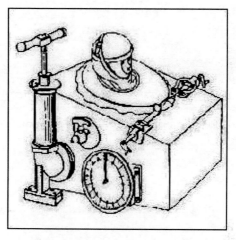

"Dum spiro spero (While I breathe, I hope)"

Anonymous

"Human subtlety ... will never devise an invention more beautiful, more simple or more direct than does nature, because in her inventions nothing is lacking, and nothing is superfluous."

Leonardo da Vinci

Pop Quiz

Most textbooks on mechanical ventilation (including this one) use hand drawn waveform graphics to illustrate various topics. Unfortunately, many authors do not pay very close attention to accuracy. While this may be excusable in some situations, it can be very confusing to those who are new to the subject and are trying to assimilate all the new ideas. It may be true that a "foolish consistency is the hobgoblin of little minds" but a careless inconsistency makes a ghost of reason.

Following are some illustrations from actual published textbooks and articles. See if you can spot the errors:

1. This first illustration has about every mistake you can make. It is supposed to show the waveforms for Airway Pressure Release Ventilation. Look at the pressure, volume and flow waveforms and pay attention to the timing. How many errors can you find?

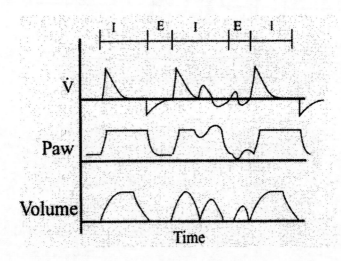

2. This illustration compares volume control with a constant inspiratory flow to pressure control with a constant inspiratory pressure. By now, it should be easy for you to see the flaws:

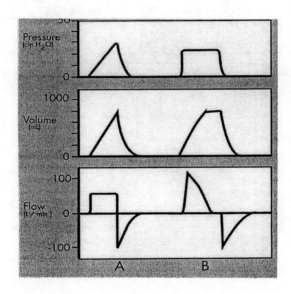

3. This illustration attempts to show the effect of normal (A) increased (B) and decreased compliance (C) during volume controlled ventilation.

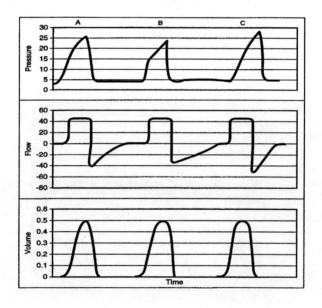

4. Here we have an illustration of the effects of increasing the pressure rise time during pressure controlled ventilation. The pressure waveforms look good but what is wrong with the flow waveforms?

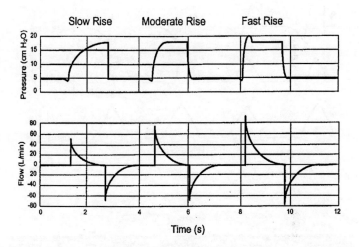

5. Finally, here is a hand drawn illustration that is supposed to show the waveforms associated with the major flow patterns produced by ICU ventilators. Compare it to Figure 5-7, which was drawn by a computer based on the equation of motion.

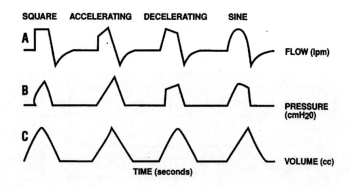

Self Assessment Questions

Definitions

- Waveform display

- Loop display

- Plateau pressure

- C_{20}/C_{dyn} index

- Dynamic Compliance

- Leak

- Pressure-time product

- Occlusion pressure ($P_{0.1}$)

- Rapid shallow breathing index

- Inspiratory force

- Work of breathing

True or False

1. The slope of a straight line is given by the equation; slope $= \Delta y/\Delta x$.

2. Constant flow into a model of the lungs with only elastance results in a triangular shaped pressure waveform.

3. If airway resistance increases and flow stays the same, peak inspiratory pressure increases.

4. During volume controlled ventilation, if compliance decreases peak inspiratory pressure also decreases.

5. During volume controlled ventilation, mean airway pressure decreases if compliance increases.

6. Mean airway pressure always changes when ventilatory frequency is changed.

7. Figure 5-3 C shows that during pressure controlled ventilation, flow decreases because volume increases.

8. During pressure controlled ventilation, if airway resistance increases peak inspiratory pressure increases.

9. For a pressure controlled breath, tidal volume decreases if airway resistance increases.

10. If a patient gets a large pneumothorax during pressure controlled ventilation, tidal volume is likely to decrease because compliance decreases.

11. Figure 5-4 shows that if resistance increases, it takes longer to achieve the same tidal volume.

12. Switching the patient from volume control to pressure control at the same tidal volume will reduce the risk of volutrauma because peak inspiratory pressure will decrease.

13. Oxygenation may be better with volume control than pressure control because volume control results in a higher mean airway pressure.

14. Plateau pressure represents the pressure in the lungs when flow is zero.

15. The pressure, volume, and flow the patient actually receives are never precisely the same as what comes out of the ventilator.

16. Patient circuit compliance can sometimes be greater than respiratory system compliance and thus have a large effect on ventilation

17. The effect of the patient circuit is more troublesome during pressure controlled modes than volume controlled modes.

18. Patient circuit compliance can cause inaccuracy in the determination of autoPEEP.

19. The area of the pressure-time curve *under* the baseline pressure is proportional to the work the patient does on the ventilator (imposed work).

20. If the pressure rise time is adjustable, and the rise time is increased, the pressure waveform changes from more rectangular to more exponential.

21. Pressure Support is a form of continuous spontaneous ventilation in which breaths are pressure or flow triggered, pressure limited, and flow cycled.

22. If there is a leak around an uncuffed endotracheal tube, more volume leaks out during expiration than during inspiration.

23. Setting the inspiratory flow high enough will eliminate the work of breathing done by the patient.

24. During pressure controlled breaths, if the inspiratory time is too short you can observe that the inspiratory flow curve is cut off prematurely.

25. AutoPEEP may be revealed on the pressure curve by using an inspiratory hold maneuver.

26. Work is represented on a loop display as the area between the volume curve and the time axis.

Multiple Choice

1. The recommended procedure for routine inspection of ventilator graphics is:

    a. Identify the mode; check the overall quality of the display, check for signs of asynchrony; check for optimal settings.

    b. Check the overall quality of the display; identify the mode; check for signs of asynchrony; check for optimal settings.

    c. Check for signs of asynchrony; check the overall quality of the display; check for optimal settings; identify the mode.

    d. Check for optimal settings; check for signs of asynchrony; check the overall quality of the display; identify the mode.

2. During VC-CMV, peak inspiratory pressure will increase if:

    a. Resistance increases or compliance decreases

    b. Resistance decreases or compliance increases

    c. Flow or tidal volume decrease

      d.   None of the above

3.   During PC-CMV, tidal volume will decrease if:

      a.   Resistance increases or compliance decreases

      b.   Resistance decreases or compliance increases

      c.   The pressure limit increases

      d.   None of the above

4.   Which of the following statements are false when comparing volume control with pressure control at the same tidal volume (see Figure 5-5):

      a.   Volume control results in a higher peak inspiratory pressure.

      b.   Pressure control opens the lungs faster.

      c.   Pressure control results in a higher peak inspiratory flow.

      d.   Pressure control should provide the lowest risk of volutrauma.

5.   A constant inspiratory pressure results in a(n) _____ flow waveform.

      a.   Exponential decay

      b.   Constant

      c.   Ascending ramp

      d.   Descending ramp

6.   A constant inspiratory flow results in a(n) _____ volume waveform.

      a.   Exponential decay

      b.   Constant

      c.   Ascending ramp

      d.   Descending ramp

7.   Examine the waveforms for DC-CMV (dual control within breaths; pressure control to volume control). If lung mechanics do not change, what would cause the switch

from pressure control to volume control to happen too soon in inspiration:

    a.   Pressure limit set too low

    b.   Tidal volume set too high

    c.   Flow set too high

    d.   All of the above

8. On a static pressure-volume curve, over-distention of the lungs is indicated by:

    a.   An upper inflection point.

    b.   The lower inflection point.

    c.   Linear compliance.

    d.   PEEP set below the optimum level.

9. All of the following are true about the C_{20}/C_{dyn} index except:

    a. C_{20}/C_{dyn} is the ratio of the compliance during the last 20% of inspiration to the dynamic compliance for the whole breath.

    b.   A C_{20}/C_{dyn} value of less than 1.0 indicates over-distention.

    c.   A C_{20}/C_{dyn} value of greater than 1.0 indicates that the pressure-volume curve cannot be used to assess over-distention.

    d.   The C_{20}/C_{dyn} index is not affected by the mode of ventilation.

10. Flow-volume loops are useful for assessing all of the following except:

    a.   Leaks in patient circuit.

    b.   AutoPEEP

    c.   Bronchodilator response

    d.   Over-distention

11. A flow-volume loop on a patient with obstructive lung disease sometimes shows an initial high flow and then a

low flow during most of expiration. This probably indicates:

    a.   Dynamic hyperinflation

    b.   Initial venting of compressed gas from the patient circuit and then flow limitation due to airway collapse.

    c.   Tidal volume is too high.

    d.   A positive response to bronchodilator treatment.

12. When comparing pre- and post-bronchodilator flow-volume loops, which of the following would indicate a positive response:

    a.   A higher peak inspiratory flow

    b.   Higher flow throughout expiration

    c.   A smaller tidal volume

    d.   Dynamic hyperinflation

13. The static method for estimating compliance uses the equation:

    a.   Tidal volume ÷ (plateau pressure − PEEP)

    b.   (plateau pressure − PEEP) ÷ tidal volume

    c.   Tidal volume ÷ peak inspiratory pressure

    d.   End inspiratory flow change ÷ (plateau pressure − PEEP)

14. The static method for estimating resistance uses the equation:

    a.   End inspiratory flow change ÷ (plateau pressure − PEEP)

    b.   End inspiratory flow change ÷ peak inspiratory pressure

    c.   (plateau pressure − PEEP) ÷ End inspiratory flow change

    d.   Tidal volume ÷ (plateau pressure − PEEP)

15. All of the following are true about the time constant except:

    a. A value of less than 3 indicates gas trapping.

    b. It is calculated as the product of resistance and compliance.

    c. After one time constant, the patient has exhaled 63% of the tidal volume.

    d. The unit of measurement for the time constant is time, usually seconds.

16. All of the following are true about the pressure-time product except:

    a. It is used as a measure of the patient's central ventilatory drive.

    b. It was originally described as an index of respiratory work or oxygen cost of breathing.

    c. When calculated with the pressure drop below baseline, it indicates the work imposed on the patient to trigger a breath.

    d. Setting the flow too low during VC-CMV will increase the pressure-time product.

17. The airway occlusion pressure is:

    a. Calculated as the pressure 0.1 seconds after the start of an inspiratory effort.

    b. Normally about 1-2 cmH$_2$O.

    c. Is relatively insensitive to changes in respiratory system mechanics.

    d. All of the above.

18. The rapid shallow breathing index:

    a. Is used when the patient is being weaned from Pressure Support.

    b. May be predictive of weaning success when it is less than 105 for adults or less than 11 for children.

    c.   Is the ratio of spontaneous breathing frequency to unassisted tidal volume.

    d.   Only b and c.

19. An inspiratory force of -35 cmH$_2$O is:

    a.   Measured by occluding the airway during inspiration.

    b.   Indicative of a greater inspiratory force than a NIF of 20 cmH$_2$O.

    c.   Predictive of weaning success.

    d.   All of the above.

20. On a loop display, work is represented by:

    a.   The pressure-time product.

    b.   The area between the pressure curve and the volume axis.

    c.   The area between the flow curve and the volume axis.

    d.   The pressure required to trigger the ventilator.

Key Ideas

1. What graphic convention is used to distinguish inspiratory from expiratory flow?

2. Describe the key differences between volume control and pressure control that can be identified on a waveform display.

3. Write the equations for calculating compliance and resistance by hand at the bedside.

4. Name the five basic flow waveforms that may be generated by modern ICU ventilators.

5. Describe the two basic types of pressure-volume loop.

6. What is an inflection point? Explain the significance of the upper and lower inflection points on a static pressure-volume loop.

7. What is the significance of the lower inflection point on a dynamic pressure-volume curve during volume controlled ventilation?

8. Discuss the problems with trying to identify inflection points on pressure-volume loops during pressure controlled ventilation.

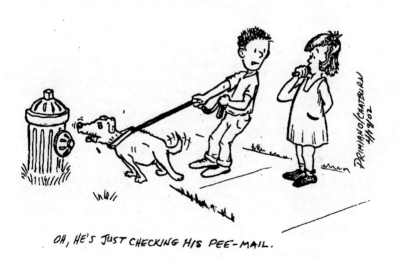

OH, HE'S JUST CHECKING HIS PEE-MAIL.

Appendix I: Answers to Questions

Chapter 1: Introduction to Ventilation

Definitions

- *Anatomical dead space:* The volume of the conducting airways in the lungs that does not participate in gas exchange.

- *Minute ventilation:* The volume of gas entering, or leaving, the lungs in a given amount of time. It can be calculated by multiplying the volume of gas, either inhaled or exhaled during a breath (called the tidal volume), times the breathing rate.

- *Tidal volume:* the volume of gas, either inhaled or exhaled during a breath.

- *PEEP:* positive end expiratory pressure. A positive pressure maintained during expiration; usually associated with assisted ventilation.

- *CPAP:* continuous positive airway pressure. A positive pressure maintained throughout the breathing cycle; usually associated with unassisted spontaneous breathing.

True or False

1. True

2. False

3. True

4. False; The unit is liters/minute

5. True

Multiple Choice

1. d

2. b

3. a Note: if you thought d was the correct answer, consider the conditions when you blow into a closed container (like a pop bottle). You can't exhale because the bottle obstructs your airway but both lung and airway opening pressure are higher than body surface pressure.

Key ideas

1. Minute ventilation determines whether breathing is producing enough gas exchange to keep a person alive. Minute ventilation is the product of tidal volume and breathing frequency.

2. The amount of carbon dioxide in the blood is inversely proportional to minute ventilation for a given level of metabolic carbon dioxide production. Therefore, blood measurements can be used to monitor the physiologic effect of ventilation. Just measuring the minute ventilation (frequency and tidal volume) does not tell whether adequate gas exchange is occurring. A normal minute ventilation may not provide adequate gas exchange if there is lung pathology or if the tidal volume is so low that only the dead space is being ventilated.

3. Positive pressure ventilators apply a positive pressure (relative to atmospheric pressure) to the airway opening. Negative pressure ventilators apply a negative pressure (relative to atmospheric pressure) to the body surface. However, in both cases, the pressure driving inspiration is positive. This pressure is called transrespiratory pressure, defined as pressure at the airway opening minus pressure on the body surface.

Chapter 2: Introduction to Ventilators

Definitions

*   *Mechanical ventilator:* an automatic machine designed to provide all or part of the work the body must produce to move gas into and out of the lungs

*   *Conventional ventilator:* ventilator that produces breathing patterns that mimic the way we normally breathe (at rates

our bodies produce during our usual living activities: 12 - 25 breaths/min for children and adults; 30 - 40 breaths/min for infants).

- *High frequency ventilator:* ventilator that produces breathing patterns at frequencies much higher than we would or could voluntarily produce for breathing (anywhere from 150 to 900 cycles per minute).

- *High frequency jet ventilator:* The HFJV directs a high frequency pulsed jet of gas into the trachea from a thin tube within an endotracheal or tracheostomy tube. This pulsed flow entrains air from inside the tube and directs it toward the bronchi.

- *High frequency oscillatory ventilator:* The HFOV typically uses a piston arrangement (although other mechanisms are used) that moves back and forth rapidly to oscillate the gas in the patient's breathing circuit and airways.

- *Spontaneous breath:* A breath for which **both** the timing and size are controlled by the patient.

- *Mandatory breath:* A breath for which **either** the timing or size is controlled by the ventilator.

- *Mode of ventilation:* A particular pattern of spontaneous and mandatory breaths.

- *Waveform display:* Waveform displays show pressure, volume, and flow on the vertical axis with time on the horizontal axis.

- *Loop display:* Loop displays show one variable plotted against another (e.g., pressure vs. volume).

True or False

1. False; a ventilator is an automatic machine whereas a manual resuscitator requires a human operator to supply the energy to ventilate.

2. True

3. True

4. False; the definition of noninvasive ventilation is that it does not require intubation with an artificial airway but rather uses a mask.

5. True

Multiple Choice

1. a

2. d

3. b

Key Ideas

1. Invasive ventilation requires the patient to be intubated with an artificial airway (tracheostomy tube or endotracheal tube). Noninvasive ventilation requires only a mask. Invasive ventilation is performed with positive pressure ventilators and noninvasive ventilation with negative pressure ventilators.

2. The distinction is important because it is the basis for defining a mode of ventilation.

Chapter 3: How Ventilators Work

Definitions

- *Transrespiratory pressure:* pressure at the airway opening minus pressure on the body surface.

- *Transairway pressure:* pressure at the airway opening minus pressure in the lungs.

- *Transthoracic pressure:* pressure in the lungs minus pressure on the body surface.

- *Transalveolar pressure:* pressure in the lungs minus pressure in the pleural space.

- *Transmural pressure:* pressure in the pleural space minus pressure on the body surface.

- *Elastance:* Δpressure/Δvolume.

- *Compliance:* Δvolume/Δpressure.

- *Resistance:* Δpressure/Δflow.

- *Total ventilatory support:* the ventilator provides all the work of breathing; muscle pressure in the equation of motion is zero.

- *Partial ventilatory support:* both the ventilator and the muscles provide some of the work of breathing; muscle pressure and ventilator pressure in the equation of motion are both non-zero.

- *Series connection:* A series connection means that two or more components share the same flow but each has a different pressure drop (the pressure difference between inlet and outlet). An example would be an endotracheal tube in series with the mainstem bronchus.

- *Parallel connection:* A parallel connection means that two or more components share the same pressure drop but different flows. An example would be the resistances of the right and left bronchi.

- *Control variable:* the primary variable that the ventilator manipulates to cause inspiration (pressure, volume, flow and sometimes time).

- *Phase variable:* a variable that is measured and used by the ventilator to initiate some phase of the breath cycle.

- *Limit variable:* a variable that can reach and maintain a preset level *before* inspiration ends but does not end inspiration. Pressure, flow, or volume can be the limit variable.

- *Cycle variable:* the variable (usually pressure, volume, flow, or time) that is measured and used to end inspiration.

- *Trigger:* to start inspiration.

- *Sensitivity:* The sensitivity setting of the ventilator is a threshold value for the trigger variable which, when met, starts inspiration. In other words, the sensitivity is the amount the trigger variable must change to start inspiratory flow.

- *Limit:* to restrict the magnitude of a variable (pressure, volume, or flow) to some preset value.

- *Cycle:* to end the inspiratory time (and begin expiratory flow).

- *Expiratory time:* the time from the start of expiratory flow to the start of inspiratory flow.

- *Expiratory flow time:* the time from the start of expiratory flow to the time when expiratory flow stops.

- *Expiratory pause time:* the time from when expiratory flow stops to the start of inspiratory flow.

- *Inspiratory time:* the time from the start of inspiratory flow to the start of expiratory flow.

- *Inspiratory flow time:* the time from the start of inspiratory flow to the time when inspiratory flow stops.

- *Inspiratory pause time:* the time from when inspiratory flow stops to the start of expiratory flow.

- *Total cycle time:* same as ventilatory period

- *Ventilatory period:* the time from the start of inspiratory flow of one breath to the start of inspiratory flow of the next breath; inspiratory time plus expiratory time; the reciprocal of ventilatory frequency.

- *Dynamic hyperinflation:* the increase in lung volume that occurs whenever insufficient exhalation time prevents the respiratory system from returning to its resting end-expiratory equilibrium volume between breath cycles; gas trapping.

- *Trapped gas:* the volume of gas associated with autoPEEP.

- *PEEP:* positive end expiratory pressure. A positive pressure (relative to atmospheric pressure) maintained during expiration; usually associated with assisted ventilation

- *AutoPEEP:* the positive difference between end expiratory alveolar pressure and the end expiratory airway pressure (PEEP or CPAP) selected by the clinician.

- *Total PEEP:* the sum of autoPEEP and intentionally applied PEEP or CPAP.

- *Mode (of ventilation):* a specific combination of breathing pattern, control type, and control strategy.

- *Volume control:* Volume control means that tidal volume and inspiratory flow are preset and airway pressure is then dependent upon those settings and respiratory system elastance and resistance (according to the equation of motion).

- *Pressure control:* Pressure control means that the airway pressure waveform is preset (for example by setting peak inspiratory pressure and end expiratory pressure). Tidal volume and inspiratory flow are then dependent on these settings and the elastance and resistance of the respiratory system.

- *Dual control:* use of both pressure and volume signals to control the breath size.

- *Dual control between breaths:* to control pressure during the breath but to control tidal volume over several breaths through automatic adjustment of the pressure limit.

- *Dual control within breaths:* to switch between pressure control and volume control during a single breath.

- *Breath:* A breath is defined as a positive change in airway flow (inspiration) paired with a negative change in airway flow (expiration), both relative to baseline flow and associated with ventilation of the lungs. This definition excludes flow changes caused by hiccups or cardiogenic oscillations. But it allows the superimposition of, say, a spontaneous breath on a mandatory breath or vice versa.

- *Spontaneous breath:* A spontaneous breath is a breath for which the patient controls the start time and the tidal volume. That is, the patient both triggers and cycles the breath.

- *Mandatory breath:* A mandatory breath is a breath for which the machine sets the start time and/or the tidal volume. That is, the machine triggers and/or cycles the breath.

- *Assisted breath:* An assisted breath is a breath during which all or part of inspiratory (or expiratory) flow is generated by the ventilator doing work on the patient. In simple terms, if the airway pressure rises above end expiratory pressure during inspiration, the breath is assisted (as in the Pressure Support mode). It is also possible to assist expiration by dropping airway pressure below end expiratory pressure (like the Exhalation Assist feature on the Venturi ventilator).

- *CMV:* continuous mandatory ventilation; all breaths are mandatory.

- *IMV:* breaths can be either mandatory or spontaneous. Breaths can occur separately or breaths can be superimposed on each other. Spontaneous breaths may be superimposed on mandatory breaths, as in Airway Pressure Release Ventilation (APRV). Alternatively, mandatory breaths may be superimposed on spontaneous breaths, as in high frequency ventilation. When the mandatory breath is patient triggered, it is commonly referred to as synchronized IMV (SIMV).

- *CSV:* continuous spontaneous ventilation; all breaths are spontaneous.

- *Pressure Support:* Pressure Support is a mode in which all breaths are patient triggered, pressure limited, and patient cycled.

- *Synchronized IMV:* IMV in which mandatory breaths may be triggered by the patient.

- *Closed loop (feedback) control:* a control scheme in which the actual output is measured (as a feedback signal) and compared to the desired input. If there is a difference, an error signal is sent to the controller to adjust the output towards the desired value.

- *Setpoint control:* the output of the ventilator automatically matches a constant, unvarying, operator preset input value (like the production of a constant inspiratory pressure or flow from breath to breath).

- *Servo control:* the output of the ventilator automatically follows a dynamic, varying, operator specified input. For example, the Automatic Tube Compensation feature on the Dräger Evita 4 ventilator measures instantaneous flow and forces instantaneous pressure to be equal to flow multiplied by a constant (representing endotracheal tube resistance).

- *Setpoint dual control:* the output of the ventilator is automatically adjusted during the breath to maintain the set tidal volume using either the set pressure limit or the set inspiratory flow.

- *Adaptive dual control:* the pressure limit of the ventilator is automatically adjusted over several breaths to maintain a target tidal volume as the mechanics of the respiratory system change. Thus, the ventilator adapts to the need for a changing setpoint. The ventilator typically monitors both exhaled volume and respiratory system elastance on a breath-by-breath basis. Then, if the tidal volume falls below the desired value, the ventilator adjusts the set pressure limit to bring the tidal volume closer to the target (required pressure change = calculated elastance x exhaled volume).

- *Optimum control* the output of the ventilator automatically matches a fixed input according to a control strategy that, as the condition of the controlled system changes, is modified optimally. Optimally means in such a way that some measure of system performance is maximized or minimized. For example, each breath is pressure limited and the pressure limit is automatically adjusted between breaths in such a way that the work of breathing is minimized and a preset minute ventilation is maintained.

- *Conditional variable:* a variable used by a ventilator's operational logic system to make decisions.

- *Operational logic:* a description of how the computer uses the conditional variables. Operational logic often takes the form of "if-then" statements. That is, *if* the value of a conditional variable reaches some preset level, *then* some action occurs to change the ventilatory pattern.

True or False

1. True

2. False; the pressure driving inspiration is transrespiratory system pressure.

3. True

4. False; the total compliance of a series connection is less than either of the individual compliances.

5. True

6. True

7. True

8. True

9. True

10. True

11. False; an inspiratory hold can only occur if the inspiratory time is longer than the inspiratory flow time.

12. True

13. False; for any variable (pressure, volume, or flow) inspiration does not end when the set limit is met. Inspiration only ends when the cycle threshold is met.

14. True

15. True

16. False; if the I:E ratio changes but the ventilatory period stays constant, frequency will stay constant.

17. True

18. True

19. False; a ventilator can control only one variable in the equation of motion (pressure, volume, or flow) at a time.

20. True

21. True

22. False; dual control within breaths requires the operator to set a pressure limit, tidal volume and flow limit and requires that these be all balanced to get the desired dual control effect. Dual control between breaths requires only the setting of pressure limit and tidal volume independently.

23. False; true CPAP maintains a constant airway pressure. An assisted breath, by definition, requires that airway pressure rise above baseline during inspiration.

24. True

25. True

26. False; feedback signals are used in closed loop control.

27. False; optimum control is the most sophisticated control strategy currently available.

28. True

29. True

30. True

31. False; a complete mode description specifies the breathing pattern, the control type, and the control strategy for both mandatory and spontaneous breaths.

Multiple Choice

1. a
2. c
3. a
4. d
5. b
6. c
7. b
8. c
9. b
10. c

11. a

12. a

13. b

14. c

15. a

16. d

17. b

18. c; the lowest work corresponds with the smallest pressure change and the largest flow change.

19. d

20. d

21. d

22. b

23. c

24. b

25. c

26. d

27. d

28. a

29. d

30. a

31. c

32. a

33. b

34. b

35. c

36. d

37. a

38. d

39. d

Key Ideas

1. *muscle pressure + ventilator pressure = (elastance x volume) + (resistance x flow)*

2. If the airway pressure rises above baseline during inspiration the breath is assisted.

3. The four variables in the equation of motion are pressure, volume, flow and time.

4. The four phase variables are: trigger, limit, cycle, and baseline.

5. *Expiratory time = expiratory flow time + expiratory pause time.*

6. During a volume limited breath, volume rises to a preset value and is held there until the breath is cycled off. During a volume cycled breath, inspiration ends the moment the set tidal volume is met.

7. *Inspiratory time = inspiratory flow time + inspiratory pause time.*

8. *Total cycle time = inspiratory time + expiratory time.*

9. If inspiratory time is longer than inspiratory flow time, then there will be an inspiratory hold. This is recognized on a graphic display as a period of zero flow between the inspiratory and expiratory flow curves. It will also show up as either a pressure or volume limit.

10. A mode is characterized by the breathing pattern, the control type and the control strategy.

11. Breaths in the Pressure Support mode are normally spontaneous because the patient can control both the timing and size of the breaths.

12. It is not very informative to say that a patient is on IMV because there are three different types of IMV; VC-IMV, PC-IMV, and DC-IMV.

Review and Consider

1. The unit of measurement that results from multiplying elastance (e.g., cm H_2O/L) by volume (e.g., L) or resistance (e.g., cm $H_2O/L/s$) by flow (e.g., L/s) is pressure. This is

confirmed by a simple dimensional analysis as shown below. It is left for the reader to do a similar analysis for the product of elastance and volume or the quotient of volume and compliance.

$$resistance \times flow = \frac{pressure}{flow} \times flow = pressure$$

$$\frac{cm\,H_2O}{L/s} \times \frac{L}{s} = \left(cm\,H_2O \times \frac{s}{L}\right) \times \frac{L}{s} = \left(\frac{cm\,H_2O \times s}{L}\right) \times \left(\frac{L}{s}\right) = cm\,H_2O$$

Thus, we see that both sides of the equation of motion are expressed in units of pressure. Pressure is defined as force per unit area. Thus, the equation of motion is an expression of the balance between the forces causing inspiration (e.g., the ventilator and muscles) and the forces opposing them (e.g., the elastance and resistance of the lungs and chest wall).

2. The equation of motion can be expressed as:

$$transrespiratory\ pressure = transthoracic\ pressure + transairway\ pressure$$

where transrespiratory pressure is ventilator and muscle pressure, transthoracic pressure is elastance times volume and transairway pressure is resistance times flow.

3. The equation for unassisted spontaneous inspiration is:

$$P_{mus} = elastance \times volume + resistance \times flow$$

The equation for assisted ventilation of a paralyzed patient is:

$$P_{vent} = elastance \times volume + resistance \times flow$$

4. For passive expiration, neither the ventilator nor the muscles generate pressure:

$$0 = elastance \times volume + resistance \times flow$$
$$-resistance \times flow = elastance \times volume$$
$$elastance \times volume = resistance \times (-flow)$$

The negative flow indicates flow in the opposite direction of inspiration, or expiration. The last equation shows that the force causing expiration is the pressure stored by the elastance of the respiratory system.

5. Compliance is the reciprocal of elastance:

$$compliance = \frac{1}{elastance}$$

Therefore, if elastance increases, (1/elastance) decreases and thus compliance decreases.

6. Using the equation

$$P_{vent} = elastance \times volume + resistance \times flow$$

we see that if resistance increases, the resistive load (resistance x flow) increases, making the right hand side of the equation increase. To maintain the equality, P_{vent} must increase the same amount.

7. The equation of motion has three variables (pressure, volume, and flow, with time an implied variable) and two constants (elastance and resistance). The form of the equation makes it clear that volume is a function of flow and pressure is a function of both volume and flow. Thus, only one variable is free to change at a time, with the values of the other two being determined by the first. This suggests that we can think of a ventilator as a device that controls any one of these variables. This leads to the natural classification of ventilators as pressure controllers, volume controllers, or flow controllers. Of course, a given ventilator may act as more than one kind of controller.

8. To determine if a ventilator was operating as a pressure controller, you would look at the airway pressure waveform. The waveform should look the same for each breath, usually somewhat rectangular. The waveform should not change as the patient changes inspiratory efforts. The flow and volume waveforms will change with patient effort.

9. If the ventilator delivers a constant flow, then it must be a volume or time cycled mode. Either way, inspiratory volume will remain constant with changing respiratory

system mechanics and patient effort. Thus, the ventilator is either acting like a volume controller or a flow controller. To decide which, you must know if the ventilator uses the volume signal to adjust the volume waveform using feedback control. If so, it is a volume controller. Otherwise, it is a flow controller.

10. The four phases of a breath controlled by a ventilator are:

      a.   Initiation of inspiration

      b.   Inspiration

      c.   Termination of inspiration

      d.   Expiration

11. There must be a defined phase variable so that the ventilator knows what to measure and when to use that measurement to switch between the different phases of a breath.

12. After a breath is delivered, the expiratory time determines how soon the next breath is delivered. For a given inspiratory time, as expiratory time decreases, ventilatory frequency increases and vice versa.

13. The expiratory time is the sum of the expiratory flow time and the expiratory pause time.

14. An expiratory hold is often manually imposed to measure autoPEEP.

15. Inspiratory time is the sum of inspiratory flow time and inspiratory pause time.

16. When inspiratory time is 1 second and expiratory time is 2 seconds, then:

$$f = \frac{1}{period / breath} = \frac{60 \text{ seconds/minute}}{T_I + T_E} = \frac{60}{1+2} = \frac{60}{3} = 20 \, breaths / minute$$

$$I : E = 1 : 3$$

$$duty \; cycle = \frac{I}{I + E} \times 100\% = \frac{1}{1+2} \times 100\% = 33\%$$

17. A ratio of 1:2 is the same as ½ or 0.50. Similarly, a ratio of 1:3 is 0.33. Thus, an I:E ratio of 1:2 is larger than 1:3. Clinicians use all sorts of vague adjectives to describe I:E ratios such as prolonged, extended, inverse, etc. To avoid confusion, just say increased or decreased.

18. When inspiratory time is longer than flow time, then there must be an inspiratory hold. This would look like Figure 3-7.

19. When you activate an inspiratory hold, you change the cycle variable from volume to time. Now the breath is both flow and volume limited because both variables reach a preset value before end inspiration.

20. When a breath is volume limited, it looks like Figure 3-7.

21. The equation of motion implies that if airway pressure rises above baseline during inspiration, the ventilator does work on the patient (work is proportional to pressure times volume). The definition of an assisted breath is that inspiratory pressure rises above baseline, indicating the ventilator does work on the patient. An ideal CPAP system is designed to hold airway pressure constant at the baseline pressure as the patient inspires. With no rise in airway pressure, there is no work done on the patient and the breath is therefore not assisted.

22. Dynamic hyperinflation is the process by which lung volume increases whenever insufficient exhalation time prevents the respiratory system from returning to its resting end-expiratory equilibrium volume between breath cycles. Trapped gas is the increase in volume associated with dynamic hyperinflation. AutoPEEP is the pressure associated with the trapped gas.

23. PEEP (applied PEEP) is the end expiratory pressure set on the ventilator. Total PEEP is the pressure above atmospheric that results from an expiratory hold maneuver when there is dynamic

hyperinflation. AutoPEEP is the difference between total PEEP and applied PEEP.

24. In Figure 3-8, device C imposes the least work of breathing on the patient. This is indicated by the lowest change in airway pressure and the largest associated inspiratory volume (area between flow curve and time axis). Remember that work is proportional to the change in pressure times the change in volume.

25. The three things you must know to uniquely describe a mode of ventilation are (1) the breathing pattern, (2) the type of control, and (3) the specific control scheme.

26. Ventilators are classified as pressure, volume, flow, or time controllers. For modes, this can be simplified because flow control implies volume control and time control is irrelevant. Thus, the three possibilities for a mode are volume control, pressure control, or switching between the two (dual control).

27. Dual control means that the ventilator uses both pressure and volume signals to control breath size. The purpose is to gain the advantage of a constant minute ventilation (from volume control) along with better patient flow synchrony while limiting peak alveolar pressure (from pressure control).

28. During "dual control between breaths", each inspiration is pressure controlled but the pressure limit is adjusted between breaths to maintain a tidal volume target. During "dual control within breaths" the ventilator switches between pressure and volume control within a breath to maintain a preset pressure limit and tidal volume.

29. A breath is defined as a positive change in airway flow (inspiration) paired with a negative change in airway flow (expiration), both relative to baseline flow and associated with ventilation of the lungs.

30. Practically speaking, the patient either retains control of the size and timing of a ventilator associated breath (spontaneous) or he does not (mandatory). Early ventilators controlled every breath. We soon learned that it was better to let the patient control as many breaths as possible. So, for both practical and historical reasons, modes are naturally thought of as patterns of the two kinds of breaths. From this simple dichotomy, three possible sequences arise (CMV, IMV, and CSV). Adding the control variable, we get eight basic breathing patterns that include all possible modes of ventilation.

31. The three possible breath sequences are continuous mandatory ventilation (CMV; all breaths mandatory), intermittent mandatory ventilation (IMV: mandatory breaths coexist with spontaneous breaths) and continuous spontaneous ventilation (CSV; all spontaneous breaths).

32. Three breath control variables (VC, PC, DC) and three breath sequences (CMV, IMV, CSV) allow for nine combinations. However, the combination VC-CSV (volume controlled continuous spontaneous ventilation) creates an inconsistency. Volume control implies that each breath is the same size. Spontaneous ventilation implies that the patient can control the size and duration of the breath. Both conditions cannot be true at the same time.

33. Both CPAP and Pressure Support are examples of pressure controlled continuous spontaneous ventilation (CSV).

34. During SIMV, mandatory breaths are patient triggered. During IMV, mandatory breaths are machine triggered.

35. Even if you knew nothing else, you know that the patient is still requiring full ventilatory support after two days. This is implied by CMV. You also know that pressure control is often used to

improve patient synchrony and limit peak alveolar pressure to reduce the risk of lung injury. You might also be aware that pressure control results in a higher mean airway pressure than volume control, for the same tidal volume and perhaps better oxygenation. Taken together, these facts should lead you to infer that the patient's condition has not allowed a quick post-op weaning and has in fact deteriorated. That is a lot of information contained in only ten letters.

36. "Assist control" usually means VC-CMV. However, strictly speaking, all it says is that the patient can trigger inspirations ("assist") or the ventilator will trigger them ("control"). That means "assist control" could also apply to PC-CMV or DC-CMV. Similarly, SIMV fails to distinguish between volume, pressure, or dual control.

37. This exercise is left to the student.

38. The Pressure Support mode is a form of pressure controlled continuous spontaneous ventilation, PC-CSV.

39. Open loop control means that the operator sets a desired output and the machine tries to achieve it. However, any environmental disturbances will change the output and the machine does not know it. On a car, open loop control would be like setting the accelerator to a fixed position. The speed of the car would stay constant only if it was traveling on flat ground. When it came to a hill, the speed would decrease going up and increase going down. Closed loop control means that the machine measures its output and compares it to the operator set input. If disturbances in the environment change the output, the feedback mechanism makes corrections. On a car, closed loop control is like cruise control. The accelerator changes as needed to keep the speed at the desired value. When the car comes to a hill, the accelerator is automatically depressed so the speed stays constant.

40. The control types listed in order of increasing complexity and sophistication are: (1) setpoint (2) servo (3) setpoint dual (4) adaptive dual and (5) optimal. This is the order shown in Table 3-3.

41. Dual control within breaths corresponds to setpoint dual control because the output of the ventilator is automatically adjusted *during the breath* to maintain the set tidal volume using either the set pressure limit or the set inspiratory flow. Dual control between breaths corresponds to adaptive dual control because the pressure limit of the ventilator is automatically adjusted over several breaths to maintain a target tidal volume as the mechanics of the respiratory system change.

42. A cynical answer to this question would be to sell more ventilators. The fact that few new modes have ever been scientifically shown to improve patient outcome tends to support this view. But most researchers would say that the ultimate goal is to provide for the patient's needs when the patient needs them. In other words, to provide just as much assistance as the patient condition warrants and to do it automatically. It is important to do it automatically because otherwise the patient will have to wait for the clinician to recognize the need and react appropriately. This requires building ever more sensing ability and artificial intelligence into the ventilator. A side effect (I am not sure if it is a benefit or not) is that the more intelligent the ventilator, the less time the clinician has to spend at the bedside making adjustments.[1]

43. Phase variables let us distinguish between mandatory and spontaneous breaths and therefore distinguish between similar modes. One

---

[1] Rose MR, et al. The effects of closed loop, autofeedback weaning approaches on therapist/ventilator interactions in the immediate post-op patient. Resp Care 2002;47(9):1061.

example might be IMV and IMV plus Pressure Support (depending on the particular ventilator).

44. The operational logic of a ventilator is a simple description of how the computer uses the conditional variables. Operational logic often takes the form of "if-then" statements. That is, *if* the value of a conditional variable reaches some preset level, *then* some action occurs to change the ventilatory pattern.

45. CMV/IMV on the Bear Cub and Bi-Level on the PB 840 are two modes that may look similar on graphics displays but may be distinguished by their phase variables (for spontaneous breaths) and operational logic are (see Table 3-4).

46. This is left as an exercise for the student.

Chapter 4: How to Use Modes of Ventilation

Definitions

- *Pressure rise time:* speed with which the peak inspiratory pressure is achieved, sometimes called pressure slope or flow acceleration.

- *Mean airway pressure:* the average pressure at the airway opening over a given time interval, or as the area under the curve for one breathing cycle divided by the cycle time (inspiratory time plus expiratory time).

- *Time constant:* The product of R and C has units of time and is called the time constant. It is referred to as a "constant" because for any value of R and C, the time constant always equals the time necessary for the lungs to passively fill or empty by 63%. For example, when the expiratory time is equal to the time constant, the patient will have exhaled 63% of his tidal volume.

- *Autotrigger:* a malfunction in which the ventilator repeatedly triggers itself because the trigger level is set too sensitive.

- *Volutrauma:* lung damage due to over expansion with too large of an end inspiratory volume.

- *Mandatory minute ventilation:* In this mode, the ventilator monitors the exhaled minute ventilation as a conditional variable. As long as the patient either triggers mandatory breaths or generates his own spontaneous breath often enough to maintain a preset minute ventilation, the ventilator does not interfere. However, if the exhaled minute ventilation falls below the operator set value, the ventilator will trigger mandatory breaths (in VC-IMV) or increase the pressure limit (in PC-IMV) until the target is reached.

- *Proportional Assist:* a unique mode that may provide the ultimate in patient synchrony. Each breath is patient triggered, pressure limited and flow cycled similar to Pressure Support. However, the pressure limit is not set at some constant, arbitrary value. Rather, it is automatically adjusted by the ventilator to be proportional to the patient's effort. The idea of this mode of ventilation is to allow the ventilator to support, and essentially cancel, the specific effects of pulmonary pathology. That is, the ventilator can be set to support either the extra elastance or the extra resistance caused by lung disease or both.

- *Automatic Tube Compensation:* This feature allows the operator to enter the size of the patient's endotracheal tube and have the ventilator calculate the tube's resistance and generate pressure to compensate for the abnormal resistive load.

True or False

1. True

2. True

3. True

4. False; minute ventilation is less stable with pressure control modes because tidal volume changes as respiratory system mechanics change.

5. False: mean airway pressure is higher for pressure control because pressure rises faster than in volume control, making the area under the pressure time curve larger.

6. False: the time constant depends only on resistance and compliance.

7. True

8. False; Assist/Control usually means volume controlled continuous mandatory ventilation.

9. False; volume control results in more even distribution of ventilation when lung units have unequal compliances.

10. True

11. False; pressure control with a rectangular pressure waveform results in alveoli opening earlier in inspiration than volume control with a rectangular flow waveform and thus improves oxygenation.

12. True; interestingly, this is not true for Pressure Support (PC-CSV) which is usually designed to make the pressure limit the set value above baseline.

13. False; PC-CMV results in a lower peak inspiratory airway pressure but if the tidal volume is the same, the peak alveolar pressure is the same and so is the risk of volutrauma.

14. True, which might not be a good thing.

15. True

16. False; spontaneous breaths between mandatory breaths lower intrapleural pressure and hence there is a lower mean intrathoracic pressure during IMV.

17. True

18. True

19. True

20. False; CPAP means constant baseline pressure so no breaths are assisted.

21. True

22. True

23. True, as with any form of CSV, not counting any form of backup mode.

Multiple Choice

1. c

2. a

3. d

4. b

5. b

6. d

7. a

8. b

9. e

10. d

11. c; the pressure control is active between mandatory breaths as either PEEP or Pressure Support.

12. a

13. e

14. a

Key ideas

1. Figure 4-1 shows that you need tidal volume and inspiratory time to calculate inspiratory flow (mean inspiratory flow = tidal volume ÷ inspiratory time).

2. European ventilators tend to emphasize minute ventilation control directly, using minute volume and rate settings, rather than indirectly using tidal volume and rate as with American made ventilators. Figure 4-1 shows that tidal volume, rate (frequency), and minute ventilation are in a mathematical relationship such that if any two are set by the operator, the third is automatically set by the ventilator. Table 4-1 shows that the equation is

   minute ventilation = frequency x tidal volume

The Siemens Servo ventilator has controls for minute ventilation and frequency. This means that tidal volume is a function of these two variables. Rearranging the above equation we get:

$$tidal\ volume = minute\ ventilation \div frequency$$

This shows that if minute volume is held constant, when frequency decreases, tidal volume has to increase.

3. Figure 4-4 shows that for the same tidal volume, both volume control and pressure control resulting in the same peak alveolar pressure. However, pressure control results in a higher mean airway pressure because the area under the rectangular airway pressure pattern (on the right) is larger than the area under the more triangular pressure pattern for volume control (on the left). Mean alveolar (lung) pressure is higher during pressure control for the same reason. Another way to look at it is that pressure control opens the lung more quickly than volume control, so lung pressure is applied for a longer time and hence mean inspiratory pressure is greater.

4. If the expiratory time is set equal to 3 time constants, 95 % of the tidal volume will be exhaled before the next breath starts.

5. During pressure controlled ventilation, if inspiratory time is only 2 time constants long, only 86.5% of the potential tidal volume will be delivered.

6. An expiratory time of 3 time constants will allow 95 % of the tidal volume to be exhaled (5 % trapped). Five time constants allow 99.3 % to be exhaled (0.7 % trapped). Thus, the amount of trapped gas avoided with an expiratory time of 5 time constants is 5% - 0.7% = 4.3 %.

7. End inspiratory volume is the sum of end expiratory volume, determined by the PEEP setting, and the tidal volume. Thus, if either PEEP or tidal volume is increased, end inspiratory volume increases.

Review and Consider

1. If the tidal volume is 0.5 L and the frequency is 15 breaths/minute, the minute ventilation is 0.5 × 15 = 7.5 L/minute.

2. If the inspiratory time is 1.0 seconds and the I:E ratio is 1:2, the frequency is

$$f = \left(\frac{60}{T_I}\right)\left(\frac{I}{I+E}\right) = \left(\frac{60}{1.0}\right)\left(\frac{1}{1+2}\right) = \frac{60}{3} = 20 \ breaths \ / \ minute$$

3. On the Siemens Servo 900c ventilator, if frequency is increased the tidal volume decreases because the operator can only set minute ventilation and frequency.

4. Mean inspiratory pressure is proportional to the area under the pressure-time curve. As Figure 4-2 shows, the area under the pressure control breath is larger than that under the volume control breath. We know this by looking at the volume/lung pressure waveforms. The area under the pressure controlled inspiration being a rectangle with one rounded edge is larger than the area under the volume controlled breath, being a triangle. The airway pressure waveforms are just these waveforms with the added pressure-time area due to airway resistance, which is the same for each type of breath. We know this because tidal volume is the same for each breath and tidal volume is just mean flow times inspiratory time. Since the inspiratory times are the same and the tidal volumes are the same then the mean inspiratory flows are the same. Mean pressure is just mean flow times resistance.

5. The time constant for the respiratory system is a measure of how quickly the system can passively fill or empty in response to a step change in transrespiratory pressure. A step change is what happens during pressure controlled ventilation during inspiration and what happens during any mode for passive expiration. Knowing the time constant helps in setting appropriate inspiratory and expiratory times on the ventilator and to predict the presence of dynamic hyperinflation. It can also be used to model volume and flow as functions of time.

6. The pressure driving inspiration during pressure controlled ventilation (pressure gradient in Figure 4-2) is the difference between peak and baseline airway pressure. Therefore, if the pressure limit is increased the pressure

gradient increases, which increases both peak inspiratory flow and tidal volume.

7. Table 4-1 gives the equation for tidal volume as a function of time. The maximum tidal volume occurs at time equal to infinity. The equation thus simplifies to:

$$maximum \ V_T = \Delta P \times C = (PIP - PEEP) \times C = (25 - 5) \times 0.4 = 8 \, mL$$

8. There are two ways to answer this question. One way is to enter the known values into the equation for tidal volume as a function of time:

$$V_T = \Delta P \times C(1 - e^{-t/\tau}) = 20 \times 0.4 \times (1 - 2.72^{-0.6/0.3}) = 6.9 \, mL$$

Another way is to recognize that the maximum tidal volume is 8 mL as shown in the previous question. Then, recognize that an inspiratory time of 0.6 seconds is two time constants. Finally, from Figure 4-4 we see that after two time constants, 86.5% of the maximum tidal volume will be delivered. Thus, 8 X 0.865 = 6.9 mL

9. The equation for mean airway pressure is:

$$\overline{P}_{aw} = k(PIP - PEEP)\left(\frac{I}{I + E}\right) + PEEP$$

From this we see that any change in I:E will change mean airway pressure. However, frequency does not appear in the equation. Therefore, if there is a frequency change that does not affect I:E, there will be no change in mean airway pressure.

10. Dynamic hyperinflation happens when the expiratory time is too short relative to the time constant of the respiratory system. Therefore, to answer this question we have to start by calculating both the time constant and the expiratory time. The equations we need come from Table 4-1. The time constant is the product of resistance and compliance:

$$\tau = RC = \frac{0.1 L}{cmH_2O} \times \frac{20 \, cmH_2O \cdot s}{L} = 2.0 \, s$$

In order to calculate the expiratory time, we first need the total cycle time and the inspiratory time. The total cycle time (TCT) is:

$$TCT = \frac{60}{f} = \frac{60\,seconds/min}{24\,breaths/min} = 2.5\,s$$

The inspiratory time is:

$$T_I = \frac{V_T}{\dot{V}_I} = \frac{0.5\,L}{60\,L/min} = 0.008\,min = 0.008\,min \times \frac{60\,s}{minute} = 0.5\,s$$

Expiratory time is thus:

$$T_E = TCT - T_I = 2.5 - 0.5 = 2.0\,s$$

So it turns out that the expiratory time for this person lasts only 1 time constant. From Figure 4-4 we see that after 1 time constant, 36.8 % of the tidal volume would be left in the lungs when the next breath occurred. Obviously, a large amount of dynamic hyperinflation is present with a trapped gas volume of 0.368 x 500 mL = 184 mL.

11. From Table 4-1 we see that:

$$P_aCO_c \propto \frac{CO_2\ production}{\dot{V}_A}$$

which says that arterial carbon dioxide tension is directly proportional to carbon dioxide production in the body and inversely proportional to alveolar ventilation. Alveolar ventilation is simply minute ventilation minus dead space ventilation:

$$\dot{V}_A = f \times (V_T - V_D) = (f \times V_T) - (f \times V_D) = \dot{V}_E - \dot{V}_D$$

We directly control minute ventilation by adjusting frequency and tidal volume. This controls indirectly minute alveolar ventilation and hence arterial carbon dioxide tension.

12. Experimental data[2] suggest that the instability of tidal volume caused by a fixed airway leak can be minimized by using pressure controlled ventilation (with a constant pressure) rather than volume controlled ventilation (with a constant flow). Either mode can be optimized in the presence of a leak by decreasing inspiratory time and increasing the tidal volume. The figure below shows the effect of a fixed leak on volume as a function of inspiratory time for pressure controlled ventilation (PCV) compared to volume (flow) controlled ventilation (FCV).

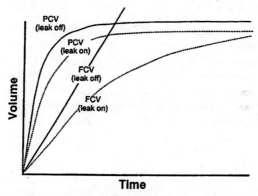

13. A patient with atelectasis and problems with oxygenation might do better with PC-CMV than VC-CMV. This is because with pressure control it is possible to open the lung earlier in inspiration (see the volume waveforms in Figure 4-3) and thus allow more time for gas exchange to occur. This early opening causes an increase in mean inspiratory pressure. That is one reason why increasing mean airway pressure often results in increasing oxygenation. Of course, increasing the I:E ratio would have the same effect. Increasing peak inspiratory pressure would have an even bigger effect. Increasing PEEP would have an effect somewhere in between changing I:E and changing PEEP.

14. The term "Assist/Control" usually refers to volume controlled continuous mandatory ventilation. However, the information contained in the term itself is only that breaths

[2] Repir Care 1996;41(8):728-735

can be either patient triggered ("Assist") or machine triggered ("Control"). Strictly speaking, this set of criteria could apply to six of the eight possible breathing patterns (VC-CMV, PC-CMV, VC-IMV, PC-IMV, DC-CMV, DC-IMV). For that reason, the term "Assist/Control" is not very descriptive and hopefully, in time, will fall into disuse.

15. This is a trick question. Peak alveolar pressure is a function of the tidal volume and the compliance. If these two factors stay the same, then peak alveolar pressure is the same for either a pressure controlled breath or a volume controlled breath.

16. Too much volume will always overstretch the lung. Too much pressure may or may not overstretch the lung. Most often, the "pressure" referred to is based on measurements made at the airway opening. A high transrespiratory system pressure (read from the ventilator airway pressure display) may be due to a high flow or resistance and thus not reflect the volumetric over-distention of the lungs. Even a high static transrespiratory pressure (a high plateau pressure) could be due to a decreased compliance of the chest wall with a normal lung distention. Therefore, the term volutrauma is more accurate than the term barotrauma. While it is true that the volumetric expansion of the lungs correlates with a high static transpulmonary pressure, the latter is almost never measured because it requires the measurement of pleural pressure (or an estimate of pleural pressure from esophageal pressure measurement).

17. Surfactant administration in the neonate often results in a short term decrease in compliance simply because of the liquid in the airways. With conventional PC-IMV, the tidal volume will decrease and gas exchange may deteriorate. With DC-IMV, the ventilator will sense this decrease in lung compliance and automatically increase the pressure limit. Later, when compliance improves, the ventilator will automatically decrease the pressure limit to and reduce the risk of volutrauma.

18. An increased level of ventilatory effort on the part of the patient is sensed by the ventilator as an increased compliance. In the DC-IMV mode, this results in a decreased pressure limit and thus a decreased level of support. If the patient has made the increased effort due to

dyspnea, he is asking the ventilator for more support but it is giving him less, thinking that he is doing better. This could lead to patient exhaustion. Of course, DC-IMV will compensate for that but the point is the patient's needs were not met at the appropriate time.

19. The difference between IMV and SIMV is that for the latter, the mandatory breaths may be triggered by the patient. In volume control, coordination with the patient's inspiratory effort is not that important in terms of tidal volume delivery. But in pressure support, mismatching between patient effort and the start of inspiratory flow can significantly decrease tidal volume.

20. CMV, implying full ventilatory support, will result in a higher mean intrathoracic pressure than IMV (implying partial ventilatory support with spontaneous breaths decreasing intrathoracic pressure during inspiration compared to mandatory breaths increasing pressure during inspiration). A higher mean intrathoracic pressure tends to decrease cardiac output.

21. Current studies suggest that IMV prolongs weaning time compared to spontaneous breathing trials or even Pressure Support.

22. Both IMV and Mandatory Minute Ventilation (MMV) guarantee the patient will receive a preset minute ventilation. The difference is that MMV can automatically switch from full support (CMV) to partial support (IM) to no support (CSV) depending on the patient's changing ability to breathe without assistance. IMV maintains the same level of support no matter what the patient does.

23. VC-IMV is indicated for patients with relatively normal lung function recovering from sedation or rapidly reversing respiratory failure. PC-IMV is indicated when preservation of the patient's spontaneous efforts is important but adequate oxygenation has been difficult to achieve with volume controlled modes.

24. PC-IMV has been used historically for neonates rather than VC-IMV because until recently, it has been technologically difficult to measure and control very small tidal volumes. One notable exception was the Bourns LS104-150 ventilator that could provide VC-CMV, VC-

IMV, PC-CMV, PC-IMV as well as CPAP. This ventilator was popular during the 1970s and 1980s but was replaced by pressure control only ventilators, probably due to cost considerations.

25. Mandatory minute ventilation using volume controlled breaths does not provide the benefits of improved patient synchrony using pressure control and may over inflate the lungs if compliance decreases. MMV using pressure controlled breaths could result in inappropriately sized tidal volumes (either too large or too small), depending on the patient's breathing rate. DC-IMV provides both improved synchrony of pressure control with the added safety of adjusting the tidal volume to be appropriate for the patient's compliance.

26. The definition of CSV is that all breaths are spontaneous. The definition of spontaneous is that the patient may control the timing and size of the breath. The definition of volume control is that the ventilator controls the size of the breath. Therefore, CSV cannot be volume controlled.

27. Although CPAP and Pressure support have the same phase variables, the pressure limit during CPAP is set equal to baseline while during Pressure Support the pressure limit is set above baseline, to provide inspiratory assistance.

28. Proportional Assist provides inspiratory assistance for both elastic and resistive loads. Automatic tube compensation provides assistance only for resistive load.

29. First, Proportional Assist is a form of CSV, so there would be no need to look up normal values for tidal volume and frequency. Second, the level of ventilatory support is set by deciding how much of the patient's elastic and/or resistive load is to be carried by the ventilator. If you think in terms of the equation of motion, other modes are set by adjusting the values of the variables in the equation (pressure, volume, and flow). With Proportional Assist, you adjust the constants of the equation (elastance and resistance).

30. The ideal mode in terms of patient synchrony (assuming the patient has a normal ventilatory drive) would provide exactly the amount of support the patient needs to overcome any abnormal lung mechanics or muscle weakness at exactly the right time. Because the patient's

need may change during a breath and from one breath to another, the ideal mode would be able to sense this need and respond immediately. That is essentially what Proportional Assist is designed to do. The only limitation, at present, is that the operator must determine and set the amount of elastic and resistive load the ventilator is to support. The ideal mode would be able to do this itself.

31. Pressure Support is often set at a low level to help overcome the resistive work of breathing through the endotracheal tube. The problem is that Pressure Support generates a relatively constant pressure throughout the breath while the real resistive load changes in proportion to the patient's inspiratory flow, which is not constant. Automatic Tube Compensation solves this problem by making the pressure generated by the ventilator proportional to inspiratory flow (actually it is proportional to flow squared as is the resistive load).

Chapter 5: How to Read Graphic Displays

Definitions

- *Waveform display:* a graphic display of pressure, volume, or flow on the vertical axis and time on the horizontal axis.

- *Loop display:* a graphic display of one control variable against another such as flow on the vertical axis and volume on the horizontal axis.

- *Plateau pressure:* the static transrespiratory pressure at end inspiration during an inspiratory hold.

- C_{20}/C_{dyn} *index:* an index of lung over-distention calculated as the slope of the inspiratory pressure volume curve during the last 20% of inspiration divided by the dynamic compliance.

- *Dynamic compliance:* the slope of the pressure-volume curve drawn between two points of zero flow (at the start and end of inspiration).

- *Leak:* the difference between the inspired tidal volume and the expired volume.

- *Pressure-time product:* The pressure-time product was originally defined as the integral of the pressure developed by the respiratory muscles (estimated using esophageal pressure) integrated over the duration of contraction. As such, it was intended as an index of respiratory work or the oxygen cost of breathing. There are many variations on this theme. For example, it may be defined as the integral of airway pressure from the time that pressure drops below baseline (during the triggering effort) until pressure crosses baseline again as flow is delivered from the ventilator.

- *Occlusion pressure ($P_{0.1}$):* the value of airway pressure 0.1 seconds after initiation of an inspiratory effort against an occluded airway. It is a measure of the patient's central ventilatory drive. Normal $P_{0.1}$ is about 1-2 cmH_2O during mechanical ventilation. Values above this indicate an increased ventilatory drive (the response of the respiratory centers to compromised pulmonary function) which may lead to exhaustion. Some data suggest that patients with $P_{0.1}$ values of 4-6 cmH_2O should not be weaned from the ventilator.

- *Rapid shallow breathing index:* the ratio of unassisted breathing frequency to tidal volume. It is an index used to predict which patients will be successfully weaned. A value of $\leq$ 105 breaths/min/L predicts weaning success in adults. In children, the threshold value is < 11 breaths/min/mL/kg where tidal volume is expressed in mL/kg body weight

- *Inspiratory force:* Inspiratory force (sometimes called negative inspiratory force or NIF) is a measure of the maximum inspiratory effort against an occluded airway after a preceding expiration. It is an index used to predict which patients will be successfully weaned. Patients with an inspiratory force of more than –30 cmH_2O are likely to succeed while those with inspiratory force of 0 to –20 may not.

- *Work of breathing:* the general definition of work is the integral of pressure with respect to volume. There are two general kinds of work related to mechanical ventilation. One kind is the work performed by the ventilator on the patient, which is reflected by a positive change in airway pressure above baseline during inspiration. The other kind is the work the patient does on the ventilator (called the imposed work) to trigger inspiration.

True or False

1. True

2. True

3. True

4. False; when compliance decreases, pressure increases (pressure = volume/compliance).

5. True

6. False; frequency may be changed without affecting mean airway pressure if the I:E ratio is held constant..

7. False; if the I:E ratio is held constant, then mean airway pressure stays constant for any frequency, assuming that the shape of the pressure waveform is not affected by the change in frequency.

8. False; if the ventilator controls pressure, the pressure waveform will remain unchanged with changes in respiratory system mechanics.

9. True

10. True

11. True

12. False; switching from volume control to pressure control at the same tidal volume will result in no change in peal alveolar pressure.

13. False; pressure control at the same tidal volume generally results in a higher mean airway pressure than volume control.

14. True

15. True

16. True

17. False; patient circuit compliance reduces delivered tidal volume more during volume control than during pressure control.

18. True

19. True

20. True

21. True

22. False; due to the higher airway pressure during inspiration, more volume leaks out during inspiration than expiration.

23. False; no ventilator setting will prevent the patient from making an inspiratory effort and thus experiencing some work of breathing.

24. True

25. False; autoPEEP is revealed by using an *expiratory* hold maneuver.

26. False; work is the integral of volume with respect to pressure, which is represented on a loop display as the area between the volume curve and the pressure axis.

Multiple Choice

1. b

2. a

3. a

4. d

5. a

6. c

7. d

8. a

9. d

10. d

11. b

12. b

13. a

14. c

15. a; this may seem tricky, the value of 3 means 3 seconds (or whatever unit of time is used for the time constant) not 3 time constants

16. a

17. d

18. d

19. d

20. b

Key ideas

1. Inspiration is indicated by flow in the positive direction; expiration by flow in the negative direction.

2. A waveform display will show volume control as having consistent volume and flow waveforms with a variable pressure waveform. Pressure control will show a consistent pressure waveform with variable volume and flow.

3. The equations for calculating compliance and resistance by hand at the bedside are:

$$compliance = \frac{tidal\,volume}{peak\,pressure - plateau\,presure}$$

$$resistance = \frac{peak\,pressure - plateau\,pressure}{end\,inspiratory\,flow}$$

4. The five basic flow waveforms that may be generated by modern ICU ventilators are exponential decay, constant, ascending ramp, descending ramp, sinusoidal.

5. The two basic types of pressure-volume loop are static and dynamic.

6. An inflection point is a region of the pressure-volume curve where the slope (compliance, $\Delta v / \Delta p$) changes. The lower inflection point of a static curve may correspond to

optimal PEEP while the upper inflection point corresponds to the volume at which over-distention occurs.

7. During volume controlled ventilation, the lower inflection point is created by the initial resistive load, the product of initial inspiratory flow and resistance. It has nothing to do with optimal PEEP, in contrast to the lower inflection point on a static pressure-volume curve.

8. Pressure control implies that airway pressure will be independent of respiratory system mechanics. Based on this alone, we would not expect to see inflection points that represent mechanical characteristics like optimum PEEP or over-distention. This is certainly true if the pressure waveform is perfectly rectangular. No upper inflection point will be observed if inspiratory pressure reaches a constant value before end inspiration. Any lower inflection point will be influenced by the resistive load and therefore useless for identifying optimum PEEP.

Review and Consider

1. The four step procedure for routine inspection of ventilator graphics is: (1) Check for the overall quality of the display; (2) Identify the mode of ventilation; (3) Check for signs of asynchrony, and; (3) Check for optimal settings and therapeutic response.

2. Inspiration is represented as flow in the positive direction and expiration is shown by flow in the negative direction.

3. The two components of peak inspiratory pressure during volume control are the resistive load (flow times resistance) and the elastic load (elastance times volume).

4. If the flow waveform during volume control is a descending ramp that goes to zero at end inspiration, then the peak inspiratory will no longer occur at end inspiration because at that time the only pressure is that due to the elastic load (flow is zero). It will not occur at the start of inspiration because the only pressure is that due to resistive load (volume is zero). It must occur sometime in mid inspiration. You can see this in Figure 5-7.

5. The area between the flow curve and the time axis is equal to volume. If the area is not the same for inspiration as expiration, there is a leak or the flow sensor is malfunctioning.

6. There is no difference. They are just two different ways of saying the same thing.

7. Increasing the pressure rise time has the effect of rounding the front edge of the pressure waveform. This means that volume now has time to accumulate before airway pressure reaches its highest value, as opposed to a rectangular waveform when pressure reaches its highest value at the start of inspiration when volume is zero. As a result, the peak driving pressure (airway pressure minus lung pressure) is reduced and so peak inspiratory flow is reduced.

8. According to the equation given in Table 4-1, it will take infinite time for tidal volume to reach the maximum value of $\Delta P \times C$. Maximum tidal volume occurs when the expression $\left(1 - e^{-t/\tau}\right)$ is equal to 1. This happens when $e^{-t/\tau}$ equals zero. Because $e^{-t/\tau} = \dfrac{1}{e^{t/\tau}}$, we see that as time, t, approaches infinity, $e^{t/\tau}$ approaches infinity and 1 divided by a number approaching infinity is a value approaching zero.

9. Just as in the answer above, it would take an infinite time for flow to reach zero for passive expiration. That is the meaning of an asymptote.

10. Plateau pressure reflects the distention of the lung (assuming a normal chest wall compliance). The assessment of lung distention by peak inspiratory pressure is distorted by the effects of flow and airway resistance.

11. Pressure controlled ventilation usually results in opening the lungs earlier in inspiration than volume control, allowing more time for gas exchange.

12. To estimate compliance at the bedside you have to measure plateau (static) pressure and tidal volume. For volume controlled ventilation, you must perform an inspiratory hold to get plateau pressure. For pressure

controlled ventilation, if flow is nearly zero at end inspiration, the pressure limit is the plateau pressure.

13. Plateau pressure in Figure 5-6 is less than peak inspiratory pressure by an amount equal to end inspiratory flow times resistance.

14. Pediatric sized patient circuit tubing is usually a lot larger in diameter than neonatal circuit tubing. This makes the compressible volume of the pediatric circuit larger and hence its effective compliance is larger. The circuit compliance could easily be larger than the patient's respiratory system compliance. This makes it difficult to control volume delivery if you try to use volume control. For pressure control, the extra compliance tends to decrease the pressure rise time which may be a problem if you need to maximize mean airway pressure for a given tidal volume and PEEP. The extra weight and size of the circuit also makes it undesirable for use with small neonates.

15. When trying to ventilate an adult with pediatric sized tubing, the problem is with the circuit resistance rather than compliance. Because the pediatric tubing has a smaller diameter than adult tubing, it offers much more resistance. This will cause peak airway pressure to be overestimated on ventilators that display pressure that is measured inside the ventilator rather than at the airway opening. The added resistance may also place a resistive load on the ventilator's flow control valve such that it delay's the response to the patient's inspiratory effort and decreases patient-ventilator synchrony.

16. From Figure 5-7 we see that changing from a constant flow waveform to a descending ramp decreases peak inspiratory pressure and increases mean inspiratory and mean airway pressures.

17. Mean inspiratory pressure is higher than mean airway pressure because mean airway pressure includes the time spent at PEEP, which lowers the average pressure over one breath. For constant pressure ventilation (Fig. 5-7 A), airway pressure is at the mean value throughout inspiration.

18. People say "decelerating flow" when they mean either a descending ramp flow waveform (volume control) or an

exponential decay flow waveform (pressure control). This term is a misnomer because flow is not decelerating for these waveforms, volume does. Flow simply decreases.

19. If a patient makes an inspiratory effort throughout inspiration during volume control, then airway pressure will be lower throughout inspiration compared to passive inspiration. This patient effort may not be evident from the airway pressure waveform.

20. The ventilator cannot tell the difference between an increase in compliance and an increase in inspiratory effort. Both look like a decreased elastic load because the ventilator only measures airway pressure and volume.

21. Dual control between breaths means that the ventilator automatically adjusts the pressure limit over several breaths in response to changes in compliance. Dual control within breaths means that the ventilator does not measure compliance but simply switches between volume control and pressure control in an attempt to maintain the set tidal volume and pressure limit.

22. Dual control between breaths requires setting a pressure limit and a target tidal volume. The actual pressure limit and tidal volume may often differ from the set values if lung mechanics are unstable. Dual control within breaths requires setting a pressure limit, a flow limit, and a tidal volume. Unlike dual control between breaths, the set pressure limit and/or tidal volume will be met each breath or else there will be an alarm regardless of lung mechanics.

23. For dual control between breaths, the actual pressure limit and tidal volume may often differ from the set values if lung mechanics are unstable. In contrast, for dual control within breaths, the set pressure limit and/or tidal volume will be met each breath or else there will be an alarm, regardless of lung mechanics.

24. When dual control within breaths is the type that switches from pressure control to volume control, the switch indicates that the pressure limit was not high enough to deliver the set tidal volume, so inspiratory time must now be prolonged until volume control can deliver the volume. When dual control is of the type that switches from volume control to pressure control, the set tidal volume

and flow were too high relative to the pressure limit, so inspiratory time must be prolonged until the set volume can accumulate under pressure control.

25. During Volume Assured Pressure Support or Pressure Augmentation (both forms of dual control within breaths where control changes from pressure to volume), if the pressure limit is set too low, then most of the breath will be volume control and the dual control advantage will be defeated. The same thing happens if the flow is set too high. If the pressure limit is set too high, then the breath will be more like Pressure Support than dual control. In addition, the inspiratory time may be too short and the peak inspiratory flow too high. If the flow is set too low, it will take longer for the ventilator to switch to volume control and when it does, the inspiratory time may end up being too long.

26. During IMV, spontaneous breaths are assisted with Pressure Support or perhaps Automatic Tube Compensation.

27. Switching from IMV to SIMV would stabilize tidal volume delivery for a neonate. This means that the size of the tidal volume would be more consistent from one mandatory breath to another.

28. Mean airway pressure would decrease if you switched from VC-CMV to VC-IMV, provided that some spontaneous breaths were present and they were assisted (if at all) at a low level.

29. When using a high level of Pressure Support in IMV, decreasing the IMV rate simply results in the patient filling in with spontaneous breaths. If those breaths are as large as mandatory breaths, decreasing the IMV rate does not decrease the level of support as expected.

30. During CSV, the pressure waveform will indicate how work is being done. Anytime the airway pressure goes below baseline during inspiration, the patient is doing work on the ventilator. When airway pressure goes above baseline during inspiration, the ventilator is doing work on the patient. During expiration, if the airway pressure goes above baseline, the patient is doing work on the ventilator (exhaling against expiratory resistance); if the pressure goes

below baseline, the ventilator is doing work on the patient (expiratory assist).

31. Increasing the pressure rise time during Pressure Support increases inspiratory flow and may increase tidal volume.

32. Peak inspiratory pressure during Proportional Assist is determined by four things; the elastic and resistive load settings and by the inspiratory volume and flow.

33. An intermittent leak most often appears on the volume waveform as inspired volume being larger than expired volume, with the waveform being abruptly reset to zero before the next breath. A continuous leak looks the same except that the flow waveform stays above zero during what would normally be expiratory pause time.

34. A pressure triggered breath shows a 2-3 cmH$_2$O drop in pressure just before inspiration (corresponding to the pressure sensitivity setting) with very little associated volume or flow change. A flow triggered breath should show less of a pressure drop but a larger volume and flow change corresponding to the flow sensitivity setting.

35. The graphic shows a mandatory volume controlled breath with a descending ramp flow waveform. The concave appearance of the pressure waveform indicates that the patient made an inspiratory effort late in the inspiratory time. However, it is inaccurate to say that the ventilator does not meet the patient demand because airway pressure stays above baseline. If the ventilator were delivering flow at exactly the same rate that the patient was trying to inhale, the airway pressure would stay at baseline. If the ventilator delivers flow at a rate lower than the patient demands, then airway pressure drops below baseline.

36. If inspiratory time is set too short during pressure control, the maximum tidal volume will not be delivered. This will be evident by a flow waveform that looks cut off, meaning it abruptly goes to zero at end expiration rather than gradually decaying to zero.

37. If expiratory time is set too short during any mode of ventilation, the expiratory flow waveform will look cut off as described in the previous answer.

38. If a patient makes an inspiratory effort during a pressure controlled breath, one of two things may happen: If the airway pressure drops but there is no appreciable flow and volume associated with it, then the exhalation manifold does not allow the patient to inspire above the flow delivered by the mandatory breath. If, on the other hand, the pressure stays relatively stable but flow and volume are generated by the spontaneous breath during the mandatory breath, then the ventilator probably has an "active exhalation valve".

39. (a) The initial high peak expiratory flow in the graphic is the gas in the patient circuit decompressing. (b) The following slow, linear flow is indicative of flow limitation due to collapsing airways. (c) Oscillations in the flow waveform usually indicate the presence of condensation in the patient circuit. (d) The abrupt transition from expiratory to inspiratory flow indicates the presence of dynamic hyperinflation.

40. Compliance can be obtained from a static volume-pressure curve by calculating the slope of a section of the curve (slope = Δvolume/Δpressure).

41. An inflection point on a pressure-volume curve is a transition from one compliance to another. One way to identify an inflection point is to draw lines through two adjacent sections of the pressure-volume curve where compliance seems to be different but constant (a straight line fits the data) the pressure at which the two lines intersect is the inflection point.

42. On a static pressure-volume curve, the lower inflection point may indicate an opening pressure (corresponding to optimal PEEP) where a large number of lung segments are suddenly recruited, thus increasing compliance. The upper inflection point represents the volume at which lung over-distention begins to occur, decreasing compliance.

43. The lower inflection point on a dynamic pressure-volume curve is the resistive load (flow times resistance). It has nothing to do with optimal lung inflation because it occurs before any volume has had a chance to accumulate.

44. Pressure control usually results in a constant pressure for at least the last portion of inspiration. A horizontal pressure-

time waveform results in a vertical pressure-volume curve. Obviously, no inflection point can be observed on a line that is constrained to be vertical.

45. The C_{20}/C_{dyn} index identifies the presence of an upper inflection point. A value of less than 1.0 indicates the possibility of over-distention. A value of 1.0 or greater is meaningless.

46. The shape of the inspiratory portion of a flow-volume loop is determined by the flow waveform delivered by the ventilator.

47. The expiratory portion of a flow-volume loop for a normal patient shows a relatively high peak expiratory flow and a nearly linear curve during expiration. A person with chronic obstructive lung disease would have a lower peak expiratory flow and either a concave curve during expiration (indicating multiple lung segments with different time constants) or perhaps a rapid drop from peak expiratory flow to a slow, linear curve indicating flow limitation.

48. A positive response to bronchodilator treatment would be indicated by an increased flow throughout expiration.

49. First, recall that the mean value of a periodic waveform is the constant value that will give the same area as the waveform over the same period. In other words, the mean airway pressure is the upper side of a rectangle whose area is the same as the pressure-time waveform. If you draw a rectangle superimposed on the inspiratory pressure waveform in Figure 5-7 B, you will get a figure that looks like this:

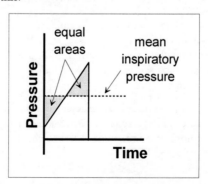

In order to make the area of the rectangle the same as the area under the pressure curve, adjust the upper side of the rectangle so that the area of the pressure curve outside the rectangle (shaded triangle on the right) is the same as the area of the rectangle outside the pressure curve (shaded triangle on left). When the two areas are equal (when the vertical heights of the two triangles are the same), the upper side of the rectangle corresponds to the mean inspiratory pressure line.

50. Mean airway pressure is determined by the shape of the pressure-time waveform (triangular, rectangular, etc), the peak inspiratory pressure, the PEEP, and the I:E ratio. It is possible to change frequency without changing mean airway pressure if the I:E ratio is held constant. In other words, the total cycle time must be changed by changing both the inspiratory time and the expiratory time by the same percentage.

51. Most ventilators use digital pressure sampling, so the calculation of mean airway pressure is simply the sum of the pressure measurements divided by the number of measurements made during the period.

52. The equations for calculating compliance and resistance by hand at the bedside are:

$$compliance = \frac{tidal\ volume}{peak\ pressure - plateau\ presure}$$

$$resistance = \frac{peak\ pressure - plateau\ pressure}{end\ inspiratory\ flow}$$

A ventilator would use multiple measurements of pressure, volume and flow (say every 10 milliseconds) and fit them with the equation of motion using regression; the constants of the equation would then be resistance and compliance.

53. The time constant is calculated as the product of resistance and compliance. If resistance is in $cmH_2O/L/s$ and compliance in L/cmH_2O, then the time constant is in units of seconds.

54. The pressure time product is an index of the work of breathing. The occlusion pressure is an index of ventilator drive.

55. The rapid shallow breathing index was developed for use with unassisted breaths. Pressure Support provides assistance and therefore may make the tidal volume higher and the frequency lower than it would be for unassisted breaths. Thus, calculating the index using Pressure Support may underestimate the patient's true value and falsely indicate weaning success.

56. An inspiratory force of −35 cmH_2O is a higher force than that which is considered minimal for successful weaning (−30 cmH_2O) although −35 is a lower number than −30.

57. Applied PEEP is the baseline pressure (relative to atmospheric pressure) set on the ventilator. Total PEEP is the pressure measured (relative to atmospheric pressure) during an expiratory hold maneuver. AutoPEEP is calculated as total PEEP minus applied PEEP and is interpreted as the pressure above baseline associated with trapped gas.

58. The work to trigger the ventilator is represented by the area of the pressure-volume curve to the left of the volume axis (pressure below baseline, volume above baseline).

Pop Quiz

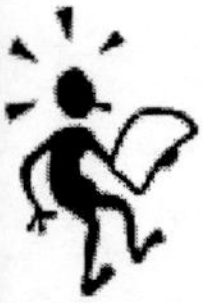

1. Starting with the top (flow) waveform, what sticks out immediately is that the inhaled volume is greater than the exhaled volume, as indicated by the area between the flow and time curves (A). Next, the shape of the inspiratory flow curves is linear, rather than exponential as it should be. The volume curve is the right shape but if you examine the time axis you see that the patient starts exhaling volume while flow is still at zero! (B)

   There is a small spontaneous inhalation and exhalation on the second mandatory breath. The pressure waveform is OK, flow is in the right direction, but a comparison of the *inspiratory* flow curve and the associated volume curve shows that the patient *exhales* the entire tidal volume! Then while he exhales, the volume appears to be inspired again (C).

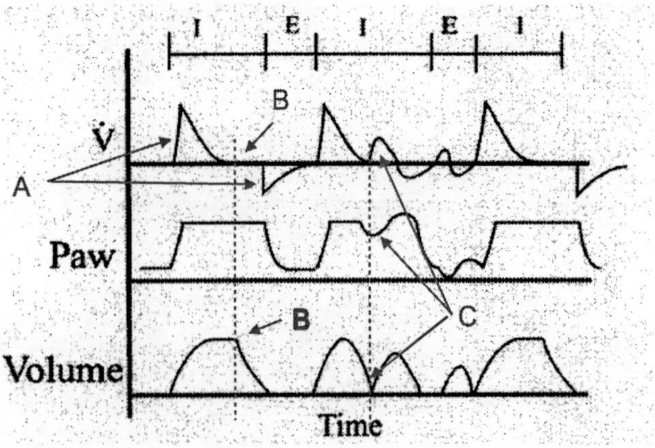

2. On the volume control pressure waveform (left) there is no initial rise due to the resistive load (A). The pressure control (right) waveforms for volume and flow should be exponential in shape but they look distorted (B). As with the previous illustration, the inhaled and exhaled volumes are different as judged by the area between the flow curve and the time axis (C).

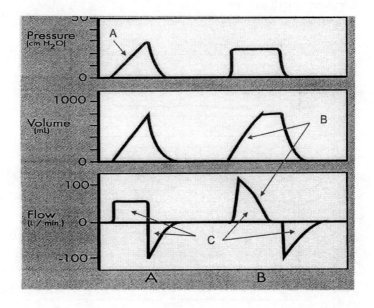

3. The initial pressure rise due to the resistive load is seen on curve B but is suspiciously absent on curves A and C. The only change was compliance, which should have changed the slope of the pressure rise as well as the peak inspiratory pressure. The volume waveforms are mysteriously rounded, when we know that a constant flow generates a triangular volume waveform. Finally, look at the volumes as indicated by the area under the flow waveforms. All the inhaled volumes are the same but the exhaled volumes are all different.

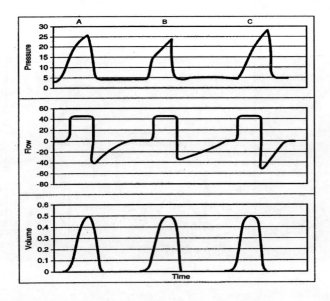

4. This illustration does a pretty good job of showing how the rise time affects the pressure waveform. The flow waveforms are correct in that they show increasing peak flow as the rise time shortens. However, the shape of the inspiratory flow is wrong. It should be rounded and peak flow should occur gradually, rather than at the start of inspiration. Even if the shapes of the flow curves were right, the inhaled and exhaled volumes indicated by the areas under the flow waveforms are not equal.

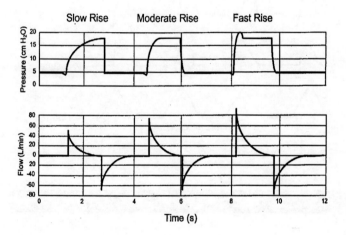

5. The first thing that catches my eye is the improper (but common) use of the terms "accelerating" and "decelerating". Aside from that, the sine flow should result in a sigmoidal rather than linear volume waveform. Intuitively, you can't have a curved flow waveform and a curved pressure waveform with a straight volume waveform.

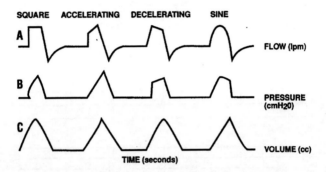

Appendix II: Glossary

Adaptive dual control: one setpoint (e.g., the pressure limit) of the ventilator is automatically adjusted over several breaths to maintain another setpoint (e.g., the target tidal volume) as the mechanics of the respiratory system change. Thus, the ventilator adapts to the need for a changing setpoint. The ventilator typically monitors both exhaled volume and respiratory system compliance on a breath-by-breath basis. Then, if the tidal volume falls below the desired value, the ventilator adjusts the set pressure limit to bring the tidal volume closer to the target (required pressure change = exhaled volume ÷ calculated compliance).

Anatomical dead space: the volume of the conducting airways in the lungs that does not participate in gas exchange.

Assisted breath: a breath during which all or part of inspiratory (or expiratory) flow is generated by the ventilator doing work on the patient. In simple terms, if the airway pressure rises above end expiratory pressure during inspiration, the breath is assisted (as in the Pressure Support mode). It is also possible to assist expiration by dropping airway pressure below end expiratory pressure (such as the Exhalation Assist feature on the Venturi ventilator).

Automatic Tube Compensation: a feature that allows the operator to enter the size of the patient's endotracheal tube and have the ventilator calculate the tube's resistance and then generate just enough pressure to compensate for the abnormal resistive load.

AutoPEEP: the positive difference between end expiratory alveolar pressure and the end expiratory airway pressure (PEEP or CPAP) selected by the clinician. AutoPEEP is the pressure associated with the trapped gas when dynamic hyperinflation occurs.

Autotrigger: a malfunction in which the ventilator repeatedly triggers itself because the trigger level is set too sensitive (sometimes mistakenly called "autocycling").

Breath: a positive change in airway flow (inspiration) paired with a negative change in airway flow (expiration), both relative to baseline flow and associated with ventilation of the lungs. This definition excludes flow changes caused by hiccups or cardiogenic oscillations. However, it allows the superimposition of, say, a spontaneous breath on a mandatory breath or vice versa.

Breathing pattern: a specific sequence of breaths (CMV, IMV, or CSV) with a designated control variable (volume, pressure, or dual control) for the mandatory breaths (or the spontaneous breaths for CSV).

C_{20}/C_{dyn} *index:* an index of lung over-distention calculated as the slope of the inspiratory pressure volume curve during the last 20% of inspiration divided by the dynamic compliance.

Closed loop (feedback) control: a control scheme in which the actual output is measured (as a feedback signal) and compared to the desired input. If there is a difference, an error signal is sent to the controller to adjust the output towards the desired value.

CMV: continuous mandatory ventilation; all breaths are mandatory.

Compliance: the constant of proportionality between volume and pressure, calculated as Δvolume/Δpressure. Static compliance is based on measurements when all flow throughout the respiratory system has ceased. Dynamic compliance was originally defined based on measurements of pressure and volume at two times when flow was zero at the airway opening (at end inspiration and end expiration). Flow may be zero at the airway opening but still present between lung units that have different time constants. The term dynamic compliance may also be extended to the technique of fitting the equation of motion to a set of pressure, volume, and flow data collected during breathing using least squares linear regression.

Conditional variable: a variable used by a ventilator's operational logic system to make decisions on how to manage control and phase variables.

Control variable: the primary variable that the ventilator manipulates to cause inspiration (pressure, volume, flow and sometimes time).

Conventional ventilator: a ventilator that produces breathing patterns that mimic the way we normally breathe (at rates our bodies produce during our usual living activities: 12 - 25 breaths/min for children and adults; 30 - 40 breaths/min for infants).

CPAP: continuous positive airway pressure. A positive pressure maintained throughout the breathing cycle; usually associated with unassisted spontaneous breathing but actually occurring during most forms of mechanical ventilation.

CSV: continuous spontaneous ventilation; all breaths are spontaneous.

Cycle variable: the variable (usually pressure, volume, flow, or time) that is measured and used to end inspiration.

Cycle: to end the inspiratory time (and begin expiratory flow).

Dual control: use of both pressure and volume as feedback signals to control the breath size. Dual control between breaths means to control pressure during the breath but to control tidal volume over several breaths through automatic adjustment of the pressure limit. Dual control within breaths means to switch between pressure control and volume control during a single breath. Control can switch from volume to pressure or from pressure to volume.

DC-CMV: dual controlled continuous mandatory ventilation.

DC-IMV: dual controlled intermittent mandatory ventilation.

DC-CSV: dual controlled continuous spontaneous ventilation.

Dynamic compliance: the slope of the pressure-volume curve drawn between two points of zero flow (at the start and end of inspiration). See Compliance.

Dynamic hyperinflation: the increase in lung volume that occurs whenever insufficient exhalation time prevents the respiratory system from returning to its resting end-expiratory equilibrium volume between breath cycles; gas trapping.

Elastance: the constant of proportionality between pressure and volume, calculated as Δpressure/Δvolume.

Expiratory flow time: the period from the start of expiratory flow to the moment when expiratory flow stops.

Expiratory hold: occlusion of the airway at the moment when the next inspiration would start in order to measure autoPEEP.

Expiratory pause time: the period from when expiratory flow stops to the start of inspiratory flow.

Expiratory time: the period from the start of expiratory flow to the start of inspiratory flow.

Flow control: maintenance of a consistent inspiratory flow waveform despite changing respiratory system mechanics.

High frequency jet ventilation: ventilation by means of a high frequency pulsed jet of gas into the trachea from a thin tube within an endotracheal or tracheostomy tube. This pulsed flow entrains air from inside the tube and directs it toward the bronchi.

High frequency oscillatory ventilation: ventilation by means of a piston arrangement (or other mechanism) that moves gas back and forth rapidly in the patient's breathing circuit and airways, causing pressure to oscillate above and below baseline pressure.

High frequency ventilator: ventilator that produces breathing patterns at frequencies much higher than we would or could voluntarily produce for breathing (anywhere from 150 to 900 cycles per minute).

IMV: intermittent mandatory ventilation; breaths can be either mandatory or spontaneous. Breaths can occur separately or breaths can be superimposed on each other. Spontaneous breaths may be superimposed on mandatory breaths, as in Airway Pressure Release Ventilation (APRV). Alternatively, mandatory breaths may be superimposed on spontaneous breaths, as in high frequency ventilation. When the mandatory breath is patient triggered, it is commonly referred to as synchronized IMV (SIMV).

Inertance: the constant of proportionality between pressure and the rate of change of flow.

Inspiratory flow time: the period from the start of inspiratory flow to the moment when inspiratory flow stops.

Inspiratory force: a measure of the maximum inspiratory effort against an occluded airway after a preceding expiration. It is an index used to predict which patients will be successfully weaned. Patients with an inspiratory force of more than –30

cmH_2O are likely to succeed while those with inspiratory force of 0 to −20 may not.

Inspiratory hold: occlusion of the airway at the moment when expiration would start in order to measure plateau pressure.

Inspiratory pause time: the period from when inspiratory flow stops to the start of expiratory flow.

Inspiratory time: the period from the start of inspiratory flow to the start of expiratory flow.

Leak: the difference between the inspired tidal volume and the expired volume.

Limit variable: a variable that can reach and maintain a preset level *before* inspiration ends but does not end inspiration. Pressure, flow, or volume can be the limit variable.

Limit: to restrict the magnitude of a variable (pressure, volume, or flow) to some preset value.

Loop display: a graphic display of one control variable against another such as flow on the vertical axis and volume on the horizontal axis.

Mandatory breath: a breath for which **either** the timing or size is controlled by the ventilator. That is, the machine triggers and/or cycles the breath.

Mandatory minute ventilation: a mode in which the ventilator monitors the exhaled minute ventilation as a conditional variable. As long as the patient either triggers mandatory breaths or generates his own spontaneous breath often enough to maintain a preset minute ventilation, the ventilator does not interfere. However, if the exhaled minute ventilation falls below the operator set value, the ventilator will trigger mandatory breaths or increase the pressure limit until the target is reached.

Mean airway pressure: the average pressure at the airway opening over a given time interval; the area under the pressure-time curve for one breathing cycle divided by the cycle time (inspiratory time plus expiratory time).

Mechanical ventilator: an automatic machine designed to provide all or part of the work the body must produce to move gas into and out of the lungs

Minute ventilation: the volume of gas entering, or leaving, the lungs in a given amount of time (usually expressed in L/minute). It can be calculated by multiplying the volume of gas, either inhaled or exhaled during a breath (called the tidal volume), times the breathing rate.

Mode of ventilation: a specific combination of breathing pattern, control type, and control strategy.

NIF: negative inspiratory force (see inspiratory force).

Occlusion pressure ($P_{0.1}$): the value of airway pressure 0.1 seconds after initiation of an inspiratory effort against an occluded airway. It is a measure of the patient's central ventilatory drive. Normal $P_{0.1}$ is about 1-2 cmH$_2$O during mechanical ventilation. Values above this indicate an increased ventilatory drive (the response of the respiratory centers to compromised pulmonary function) which may lead to exhaustion. Some data suggest that patients with $P_{0.1}$ values of 4-6 cmH$_2$O should not be weaned from the ventilator.

Operational logic: a description of how the computer uses the conditional variables. Operational logic often takes the form of "if-then" statements. That is, *if* the value of a conditional variable reaches some preset level, *then* some action occurs to change the ventilatory pattern.

Optimum control: automatic adjustment of setpoints to optimize other variables as respiratory mechanics change. The term optimum implies that some measure of system performance is maximized or minimized. For example, each breath is pressure limited and the pressure limit is automatically adjusted between breaths in such a way that the work of breathing is minimized and a preset minute ventilation is maintained.

Parallel connection: a connection in which two or more components share the same pressure drop but different flows. An example would be the resistances of the right and left bronchi.

Partial ventilatory support: both the ventilator and the muscles provide some of the work of breathing; muscle pressure and ventilator pressure in the equation of motion are both non-zero.

PC-CMV: pressure controlled continuous mandatory ventilation.

PC-IMV: pressure controlled intermittent mandatory ventilation.

PC-CSV: pressure controlled continuous spontaneous ventilation.

PEEP: positive end expiratory pressure. A positive pressure (relative to atmospheric pressure) maintained during expiration; usually associated with assisted ventilation.

Phase: one of four significant events that occur during a ventilatory cycle: (1) the change from expiration to inspiration, (2) inspiration, (3) the change from inspiration to expiration, and (4) expiration.

Phase variable: a variable that is measured and used by the ventilator to initiate some phase of the breath cycle.

Plateau pressure: the static transrespiratory pressure at end inspiration during an inspiratory hold.

Pressure control: maintenance of a consistent transrespiratory pressure waveform despite changing respiratory system mechanics.

Pressure rise time: speed with which the peak inspiratory pressure is achieved, sometimes called pressure slope or flow acceleration.

Pressure Support: Pressure Support is a mode in which all breaths are patient triggered, pressure limited, and patient cycled.

Pressure-time product: The pressure-time product was originally defined as the integral of the pressure developed by the respiratory muscles (estimated using esophageal pressure) integrated over the duration of contraction. As such, it was intended as an index of respiratory work or the oxygen cost of breathing. There are many variations on this theme. For example, it may be defined as the integral of airway pressure from the time that pressure drops below baseline (during the triggering effort) until pressure crosses baseline again as flow is delivered from the ventilator.

Proportional Assist: a unique mode that may provide the ultimate in patient synchrony. Each breath is patient triggered, pressure limited and flow cycled similar to Pressure Support. However, the pressure limit is not set at some constant, arbitrary value. Rather, it is automatically adjusted by the ventilator to be proportional to the patient's effort. The idea of this mode of ventilation is to allow the ventilator to support, and essentially cancel, the specific effects of pulmonary pathology. That is, the ventilator can be set to support either the extra elastance or the extra resistance caused by lung disease or both.

Rapid shallow breathing index: the ratio of unassisted breathing frequency to tidal volume. It is an index used to predict which patients will be successfully weaned. A value of $\leq$ 105 breaths/min/L predicts weaning success in adults. In children, the threshold value is < 11 breaths/min/mL/kg where tidal volume is expressed in mL/kg body weight

Resistance: the constant of proportionality between pressure and flow: Δpressure/Δflow.

Sensitivity: The sensitivity setting of the ventilator is a threshold value for the trigger variable which, when met, starts inspiration. In other words, the sensitivity is the amount the trigger variable must change to start inspiratory flow.

Series connection: A series connection means that two or more components share the same flow but each has a different pressure drop (the pressure difference between inlet and outlet). An example would be an endotracheal tube in series with the mainstem bronchus.

Servo control: the output of the ventilator automatically follows a dynamic, varying, operator specified input. For example, the Automatic Tube Compensation feature on the Dräger Evita 4 ventilator measures instantaneous flow and forces instantaneous pressure to be equal to flow multiplied by a constant (representing endotracheal tube resistance).

Setpoint control: the output of the ventilator automatically matches a constant, unvarying, operator preset input value (like the production of a constant inspiratory pressure or flow from breath to breath).

Setpoint dual control: the output of the ventilator is automatically adjusted during the breath to maintain the set tidal volume using either the set pressure limit or the set inspiratory flow.

Spontaneous breath: A breath for which **both** the timing and size are controlled by the patient. That is, the patient both triggers and cycles the breath.

Synchronized IMV: IMV in which mandatory breaths may be triggered by the patient.

Tidal volume: the volume of gas, either inhaled or exhaled, during a breath.

Time constant: the time at which an exponential function attains 63% of its steady state value in response to a step input; the time necessary for the lungs to passively empty by 63% or to passively fill 63% during pressure controlled ventilation with a rectangular pressure waveform. The time constant is calculated as the product of resistance and compliance.

Total cycle time: same as ventilatory period, the sum of inspiratory time and expiratory time.

Total PEEP: the sum of autoPEEP and intentionally applied PEEP or CPAP.

Total ventilatory support: the ventilator provides all the work of breathing; muscle pressure in the equation of motion is zero.

Transairway pressure: pressure at the airway opening minus pressure in the lungs.

Transalveolar pressure: pressure in the lungs minus pressure in the pleural space.

Transmural pressure: pressure in the pleural space minus pressure on the body surface.

Transpulmonary pressure: pressure at the airway opening minus pressure in the pleural space.

Transrespiratory pressure: pressure at the airway opening minus pressure on the body surface.

Transthoracic pressure: pressure in the lungs minus pressure on the body surface.

Trapped gas: the volume of gas associated with autoPEEP (see dynamic hyperinflation)

Trigger: to start inspiration.

Ventilatory period: the time from the start of inspiratory flow of one breath to the start of inspiratory flow of the next breath; inspiratory time plus expiratory time; the reciprocal of ventilatory frequency.

Volume control: maintenance of a consistent inspiratory volume waveform despite changing respiratory system mechanics, using feedback control with the volume signal.

VC-CMV: volume controlled continuous mandatory ventilation.

VC-IMV: volume controlled intermittent mandatory ventilation.

Volutrauma: lung damage due to over expansion with too large of an end inspiratory volume.

Waveform display: a graphic display of pressure, volume, or flow on the vertical axis and time on the horizontal axis.

Work of breathing: the general definition of work is the integral of pressure with respect to volume. There are two general kinds of work related to mechanical ventilation. One kind is the work performed by the ventilator on the patient, which is reflected by a positive change in airway pressure above baseline during inspiration. The other kind is the work the patient does on the ventilator (called the imposed work) to trigger inspiration.

Appendix III: Mode Concordance

This table shows the correspondence between the names of common modes with their breathing pattern classifications. A more detailed description of the modes, including control type, phase variables and operational logic may be obtained by reading the specific ventilator's operator and service manuals.

Manufacturer	Model	Manufacturer's Mode Name	Breathing Pattern
Cardiopulmonary	Venturi	Continuous positive airway pressure	PC-CSV
Cardiopulmonary	Venturi	Pressure control assist control	PC-CMV
Cardiopulmonary	Venturi	Pressure control synchronized intermittent mandatory ventilation	PC-IMV
Cardiopulmonary	Venturi	Variable pressure control	DC-CMV
Cardiopulmonary	Venturi	Variable pressure support	DC-CSV
Cardiopulmonary	Venturi	Volume control assist control	VC-CMV
Cardiopulmonary	Venturi	Volume control synchronized intermittent mandatory ventilation	VC-IMV
Dräger	Babylog	Assist/control	PC-CMV
Dräger	Babylog	Continuous positive airway pressure	PC-CSV
Dräger	Babylog	Synchronized intermittent mandatory ventilation	PC-IMV
Dräger	Evita 4	Airway pressure release ventilation	PC-IMV
Dräger	Evita 4	Automatic tube compensation	PC-CSV
Dräger	Evita 4	Continuous mandatory ventilation	VC-CMV
Dräger	Evita 4	Continuous mandatory ventilation + assist	VC-CMV
Dräger	Evita 4	Continuous mandatory ventilation + autoflow	DC-CMV
Dräger	Evita 4	Continuous mandatory ventilation + pressure limited ventilation	DC-CMV
Dräger	Evita 4	Continuous positive airway pressure	PC-CSV
Dräger	Evita 4	Mandatory minute volume ventilation + autoflow	DC-IMV
Dräger	Evita 4	Mandatory minute volume ventilation + pressure limited ventilation	DC-IMV
Dräger	Evita 4	Mandatory minute volume ventilation + pressure support	VC-IMV

Mechanical Ventilation

Manufacturer	Model	Manufacturer's Mode Name	Breathing Pattern
Dräger	Evita 4	Pressure controlled ventilation + (bi-level positive airway pressure) /pressure support	PC-IMV
Dräger	Evita 4	Pressure controlled ventilation + assist	PC-CMV
Dräger	Evita 4	Pressure support	PC-CSV
Dräger	Evita 4	Synchronized intermittent mandatory ventilation + autoflow	DC-IMV
Dräger	Evita 4	Synchronized intermittent mandatory ventilation + pressure limited ventilation	DC-IMV
Dräger	Evita 4	Synchronized intermittent mandatory ventilation + pressure support	VC-IMV
Hamilton	Galileo	Adaptive Support Ventilation	DC-IMV
Hamilton	Galileo	Assist Control (Synchronized Controlled Mandatory Ventilation)	VC-CMV
Hamilton	Galileo	Pressure-Controlled Assist Control (Pressure-Controlled, Controlled Mandatory Ventilation)	PC-CMV
Hamilton	Galileo	Pressure-Controlled Assist Control (Pressure-Controlled, Controlled Mandatory Ventilation) + Adaptive Pressure Ventilation	DC-CMV
Hamilton	Galileo	Pressure-Controlled Synchronized Intermittent Mandatory Ventilation	PC-IMV
Hamilton	Galileo	Pressure-Controlled Synchronized Intermittent Mandatory Ventilation + Pressure Support	PC-IMV
Hamilton	Galileo	Pressure-Controlled Synchronized Intermittent Mandatory Ventilation + Adaptive Pressure Ventilation	DC-IMV
Hamilton	Galileo	Spontaneous	PC-CSV
Hamilton	Galileo	Synchronized Intermittent Mandatory Ventilation	VC-IMV
Hamilton	Galileo	Synchronized Intermittent Mandatory Ventilation + Pressure Support	VC-IMV
Newport	Breeze	Pressure control assist control	PC-CMV
Newport	Breeze	Pressure control synchronized intermittent mandatory ventilation	PC-IMV
Newport	Breeze	Spontaneous	PC-CSV
Newport	Breeze	Volume control assist control	VC-CMV
Newport	Breeze	Volume control synchronized intermittent mandatory ventilation	VC-IMV

Manufacturer	Model	Manufacturer's Mode Name	Breathing Pattern
Newport	E100i	Assist/control	VC-CMV
Newport	E100i	Synchronized intermittent mandatory ventilation	VC-IMV
Newport	E100i	Spontaneous	PC-CSV
Newport	Wave	Assist/control	PC-CMV
Newport	Wave	Spontaneous + pressure support	PC-CSV
Newport	Wave	Synchronized intermittent mandatory ventilation	PC-IMV
Puritan Bennett	7200	Continuous mechanical ventilation	VC-CMV
Puritan Bennett	7200	Continuous mechanical ventilation + pressure control	PC-CMV
Puritan Bennett	7200	Continuous positive airway pressure + pressure support	PC-CSV
Puritan Bennett	7200	Synchronized intermittent mandatory ventilation	VC-IMV
Puritan Bennett	7200	Synchronized intermittent mandatory ventilation+ pressure control	PC-IMV
Puritan Bennett	740	Assist/control	VC-CMV
Puritan Bennett	740	Continuous positive airway pressure + pressure support	PC-CSV
Puritan Bennett	740	Synchronized intermittent mandatory ventilation	VC-IMV
Puritan Bennett	840	Bi-level	PC-IMV
Puritan Bennett	840	Pressure control assist control	PC-CMV
Puritan Bennett	840	Pressure control synchronized intermittent mandatory ventilation	PC-IMV
Puritan Bennett	840	Spontaneous	PC-CSV
Puritan Bennett	840	Synchronized intermittent mandatory ventilation	VC-IMV
Puritan Bennett	840	Tube compensation	PC-CSV
Puritan Bennett	840	Volume control assist control	VC-CMV
Puritan Bennett	Infant Star	Continuous flow intermittent mandatory ventilation	PC-IMV
Puritan Bennett	Infant Star	Continuous positive airway pressure	PC-CSV
Puritan Bennett	Infant Star	Demand flow intermittent mandatory ventilation	PC-IMV
Sechrist	IV-100B	Continuous positive airway pressure	PC-CSV
Sechrist	IV-100B	Ventilation	PC-IMV
Sechrist	IV-200 SAVI	Continuous positive airway pressure	PC-CSV
Sechrist	IV-200 SAVI	Ventilation	PC-IMV

Mechanical Ventilation

Manufacturer	Model	Manufacturer's Mode Name	Breathing Pattern
Sechrist	IV-200 SAVI	Ventilation + patient trigger	PC-CMV
Siemens	Servo 300	Pressure control	PC-CMV
Siemens	Servo 300	Pressure regulated volume control	DC-CMV
Siemens	Servo 300	Pressure support/continuous positive airway pressure	PC-CSV
Siemens	Servo 300	Synchronized intermittent mandatory ventilation (pressure control) + pressure support	PC-IMV
Siemens	Servo 300	Synchronized intermittent mandatory ventilation (volume control) + pressure support	VC-IMV
Siemens	Servo 300	Volume control	VC-CMV
Siemens	Servo 300	Volume support	DC-CSV
Siemens	Servo 900	Continuous positive airway pressure	PC-CSV
Siemens	Servo 900	Pressure control	PC-CMV
Siemens	Servo 900	Pressure support	PC-CSV
Siemens	Servo 900	Synchronized intermittent mandatory ventilation	VC-IMV
Siemens	Servo 900	Volume control	VC-CMV
Viasys	Bear 1000	Assist control mechanical ventilation	VC-CMV
Viasys	Bear 1000	Assist control mechanical ventilation + pressure augment	DC-IMV
Viasys	Bear 1000	Minimum minute volume	VC-IMV
Viasys	Bear 1000	Pressure control	PC-CMV
Viasys	Bear 1000	Pressure support/continuous positive airway pressure	PC-CSV
Viasys	Bear 1000	Synchronized intermittent mandatory ventilation + pressure augment	DC-IMV
Viasys	Bear 1000	Synchronized intermittent mandatory ventilation + pressure support	VC-IMV
Viasys	Bear Cub 750	Assist/control	VC-CMV

Manufacturer	Model	Manufacturer's Mode Name	Breathing Pattern
Viasys	Bear Cub 750	Assist/control	PC-CMV
Viasys	Bear Cub 750	Continuous positive airway pressure	PC-CSV
Viasys	Bear Cub 750	Intermittent mandatory ventilation	VC-IMV
Viasys	Bear Cub 750	Intermittent mandatory ventilation	PC-IMV
Viasys	Bird 8400ST	Assist/control	VC-CMV
Viasys	Bird 8400ST	Continuous positive airway pressure + pressure support	PC-CSV
Viasys	Bird 8400ST	Synchronized intermittent mandatory ventilation	VC-IMV
Viasys	Bird T Bird	Assist/control	VC-CMV
Viasys	Bird T Bird	Assist/control + pressure control	PC-CMV
Viasys	Bird T Bird	Assist/control + volume assured pressure support	DC-CMV
Viasys	Bird T Bird	Continuous positive airway pressure + pressure support	PC-CSV
Viasys	Bird T Bird	Intermittent mandatory ventilation	VC-IMV
Viasys	Bird T Bird	Intermittent mandatory ventilation + pressure support	PC-IMV
Viasys	Bird T Bird	Intermittent mandatory ventilation + volume assured pressure support	DC-IMV
Viasys	Bird V.I.P.	Continuous positive airway pressure	PC-CSV
Viasys	Bird V.I.P.	Time cycled assist control	PC-CMV
Viasys	Bird V.I.P.	Time cycled intermittent mandatory ventilation	PC-IMV
Viasys	Bird V.I.P.	Volume cycled assist control	VC-CMV
Viasys	Bird V.I.P.	Volume cycled intermittent mandatory ventilation	VC-IMV

Index

M

Machine, 7, 17, 221, 277
Machine cycled, 35
Mandatory breath
  definition, 49, 227
Mandatory Minute
  Ventilation, 59, 71, 105,
  108, 251
Mechanical ventilator, 7
Mechanics
  linear regression
    technique, 195, 198
  static vs dynamic, 192,
    194
Minute ventilation, 1
Mode
  definition, 11, 41
  specification, 42, 58
Model, 19, 283
  multi-compartment, 22
  respiratory system, 19, 20
Muscles, of respiration, 2, 5

O

Operational logic, 58, 80,
  241
Optimum PEEP, 178
Over-distention, 180, 215
Oxygenation, 98, 99, 106,
  178, 251

P

Parallel connection, 24, 224
  lungs, 132
  patient circuit and
    respiratory system, 140
Partial ventilatory support,
  21, 99, 107, 115, 118, 251
Patient circuit
  definition, 9

effects, 138, 212
resistance and
  compliance, 22
Patient cycled, 35
PEEP
  history, 3
PEP, 37
Phase variable, 28, 57
P_{max}, 46, 47, 107, 154
Pressure
  airway occlusion, 201
  mean airway, defined, 88,
    190
  muscle, 20, 147
  plateau, 136, 195
  transairway, 20, 22, 25,
    135, 136, 193, 233
  transalveolar, 24, 100,
    135, 136
  transmural, 25, 136
  transpulmonary, 20, 25,
    250
  transrespiratory, 19
  transthoracic, 20, 24, 25,
    69, 135, 136, 193, 233
Pressure Augment, 44, 53,
  153
Pressure control
  definition, 43
Pressure Controlled Inverse
  Ratio Ventilation, 100
Pressure controller, 26
Pressure Limited
  Ventilation, 53
Pressure Regulated Volume
  Control, 54
Pressure rise time, 84, 151,
  162, 212
Pressure Support, 33, 46,
  58, 109, 162, 204, 213,
  227, 279

Order Form

Email orders: rlc6@po.cwru.edu

Postal orders:
> Mandu Press Ltd.
> PO Box 18284
> Cleveland Heights, OH   44118-0288, USA

Please send _____copies of *Fundamentals of Mechanical Ventilation* for **$59.95** each to the address below.

Sales Tax: Please add 7% for orders shipped to Ohio addresses.

Shipping by air
  US: $4.00 for first book or disk and $2.00 for each additional item.

  International: $9.00 for first book or disk and $5.00 for each additional item (estimate).

Payments must accompany order. Allow 3 weeks for delivery.

Name: _____

Address: _____

_____

City: _____ **State:** _____ **Zip** _____

Telephone: _____

Email address: _____